Massage
Total Relaxation

Fitness, Health & Nutrition was created by Rebus, Inc. and published by Time-Life Books.

REBUS, INC.

Publisher: RODNEY FRIEDMAN

Editor: CHARLES L. MEE JR.
Executive Editor: THOMAS DICKEY
Managing Editor: SUSAN BRONSON
Senior Editor: MARY CROWLEY
Associate Editors: WILLIAM DUNNETT, CARL LOWE
Contributing Editors: JACQUELINE DAMIAN,
FELICIA HALPERT, LINDA HELLER

Art Director: JUDITH HENRY
Designer: DEBORAH RAGASTO
Photographer: STEVEN MAYS
Photo Stylist: NOLA LOPEZ
Photo Assistant: TIMOTHY JEFFS

Test Kitchen Director: GRACE YOUNG
Contributing Editor: MARYA DALRYMPLE
Recipe Editor: BONNIE J. SLOTNICK
Nutritional Analyst: HILL NUTRITION ASSOCIATES

Chief of Research: CARNEY MIMMS
Assistant Editor: JACQUELINE DILLON

Time-Life Books Inc. is a wholly owned subsidiary of
TIME INCORPORATED

Founder: HENRY R. LUCE 1898-1967

Editor-in-Chief: HENRY ANATOLE GRUNWALD
Chairman and Chief Executive Officer: J. RICHARD MUNRO
President and Chief Operating Officer: N.J. NICHOLAS JR.
Chairman of the Executive Committee: RALPH P. DAVIDSON
Corporate Editor: RAY CAVE
Executive Vice President, Books: KELSO F. SUTTON
Vice President, Books: GEORGE ARTANDI

TIME-LIFE BOOKS INC.

Editor: GEORGE CONSTABLE

Executive Editor: ELLEN PHILLIPS
Director of Design: LOUIS KLEIN
Director of Editorial Resources: PHYLLIS K. WISE
Editorial Board: RUSSELL B. ADAMS JR., DALE M. BROWN,
ROBERTA CONLAN, THOMAS H. FLAHERTY, LEE HASSIG,
DONIA ANN STEELE, ROSALIND STUBENBERG, KIT VAN
TULLEKEN, HENRY WOODHEAD
Director of Photography and Research: JOHN CONRAD
WEISER

President: CHRISTOPHER T. LINEN
Chief Operating Officer: JOHN M. FAHEY JR.
Senior Vice Presidents: JAMES L. MERCER,
LEOPOLDO TORALBALLA
Vice Presidents: STEPHEN L. BAIR, RALPH J. CUOMO,
NEAL GOFF, STEPHEN L. GOLDSTEIN, JUANITA T. JAMES,
HALLETT JOHNSON III, CAROL KAPLAN, SUSAN J.
MARUYAMA, ROBERT H. SMITH, PAUL R. STEWART,
JOSEPH J. WARD
Director of Production Services: ROBERT J. PASSANTINO

Editorial Operations
Copy Chief: DIANE ULLIUS
Editorial Operations: CAROLINE A. BOUBIN (MANAGER)
Production: CELIA BEATTIE
Library: LOUISE D. FORSTALL

FITNESS, HEALTH & NUTRITION

Massage
Total Relaxation

Time-Life Books, Alexandria, Virginia

CONSULTANTS FOR THIS BOOK

Marquetta K. Hungerford, Ph.D., is a codirector of the Sports Massage Training Institute and Dean and President of the American Institute of Massage Therapy, both in Costa Mesa, Calif. Hungerford, who holds doctorates in both physical therapy and nutrition, was instrumental in making sports massage available to participants in the 1984 Olympic Games in Los Angeles. She is also a consultant to the Sports Massage Division of the American Massage Therapy Association, as well as the former national director of education for the American Massage Therapy Association.

Ann Grandjean, M.S., is Associate Director of the Swanson Center for Nutrition, Omaha, Neb.; chief nutrition consultant to the U.S. Olympic Committee; and an instructor in the Sports Medicine Porgram, Orthopedic Surgery Department, University of Nebraska Medical Center.

Myron Winick, M.D., is the R.R. Williams Professor of Nutrition, Professor of Pediatrics, Director of the Institute of Human Nutrition, and Director of the Center for Nutrition, Genetics and Human Development at Columbia University College of Physicians and Surgeons. He has served on the Food and Nutrition Board of the National Academy of Sciences and is the author of many books, including *Your Personalized Health Profile*.

The following consultants helped design the massage sequences in this book:

Kenneth A. Allwood, a licensed massage therapist specializing in sports massage, is a cofounder of the American Institute of Sports Massage. A graduate of the Sports Massage Training Institute in Costa Mesa, Calif., and the Swedish Institute of Massage in New York City, Allwood teaches anatomy, physiology, pathology and medical massage at the Swedish Institute.

Russ Borner, a former executive with AT&T, is a licensed massage therapist and a cofounder and president of International Health Systems, which provides on-site massage to corporate personnel, as well as stress-management workshops and seminars.

Harry R. Elden, Ph.D., is a licensed massage therapist and a clinical investigator and biophysics laboratory director for studies on aging. He has served as a consultant to the Howard Hughes Medical Institute, the National Institute of Aging and the Xienta Institute for Skin Research in Bernville, Pa.

Laura Norman, M.S., is a registered certified reflexologist and licensed massage therapist. The founder and director of the most extensive reflexology center in the U.S., Norman developed a reflexology-training program that is offered at New York University's Division of Nursing, the Swedish Institute of Massage in New York City and other institutions.

Elaine Stillerman is a licensed massage therapist in New York City and vice president of the Alliance of Massage Therapists. A former instructor at the Swedish Institute for Massage in New York City, Stillerman has conducted numerous workshops on massage.

For information about any Time-Life book please write:
Reader Information
Time-Life Customer Service
P.O. Box C-32068
Richmond, Virginia 23261-2068

First printing.
Published simultaneously in Canada.
School and library distribution by Silver Burdett Company, Morristown, New Jersey.

TIME-LIFE is a trademark of Time Incorporated U.S.A.

Library of Congress Cataloging-in-Publication Data
Massage: total relaxation.
(Fitness, health & nutrition)
Includes index.
1. Massage. 2. Massage–Psychological aspects. I. Time-Life Books.
II. Series: Fitness, health and nutrition.
RA780.5.M37 1987   615.8'22   87-10175
ISBN 0-8094-6175-7
ISBN 0-8094-6176-5 (lib. bdg.)

This book is not intended as a substitute for the advice of a physician. Readers who have, or suspect they may have, specific medical problems, especially those involving their muscles and joints, are urged to consult a physician before beginning any massage program.

CONTENTS

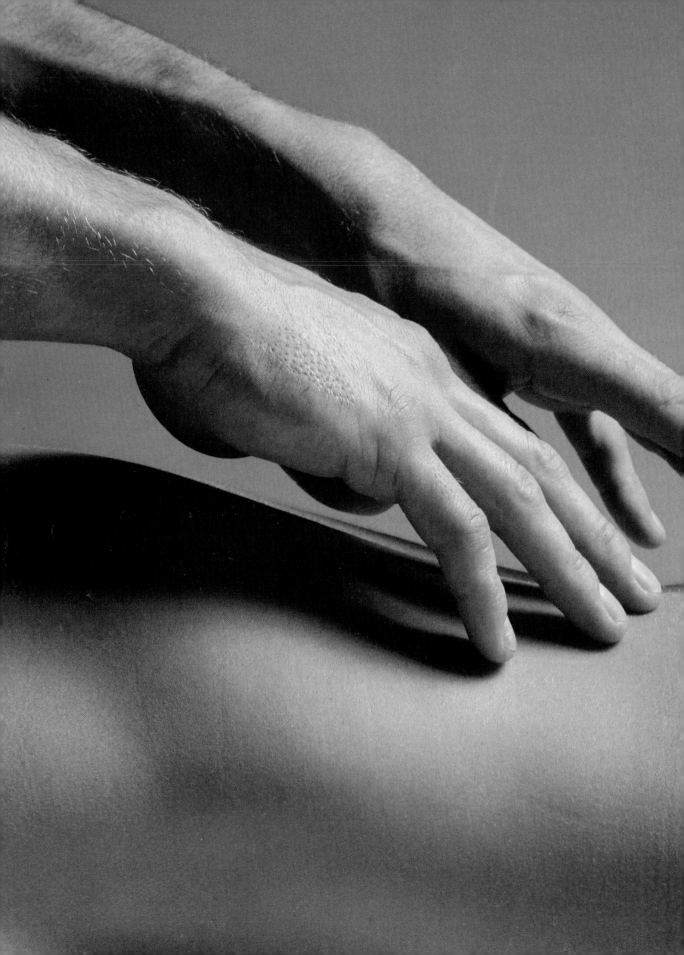

CHAPTER ONE

What Massage Can Do

Techniques of touch for promoting relaxation, keeping muscles flexible and preventing injury

Anyone who has had a good back rub knows that being stroked is a soothing and pleasurable way to unwind. But a thorough, skillfully administered massage is more than just a wonderful means of pampering yourself or a partner. The relaxation that a massage induces is physiological as well as mental, affecting nearly every system of the body. Massage can relieve stress, alleviate pain, flush toxins from tired muscles and help prevent injuries. Because its benefits have become more widely recognized, physical therapists are increasingly incorporating massage into muscular rehabilitation. Athletes are also using massage more extensively; for example, the U.S. Olympic Committee made massage available for the first time to some participants in the 1984 Olympic Games. Virtually anyone can learn to give an effective massage, so that massage can become part of a general fitness program — a component that, like exercising and eating right, helps you maintain and improve your body's functioning.

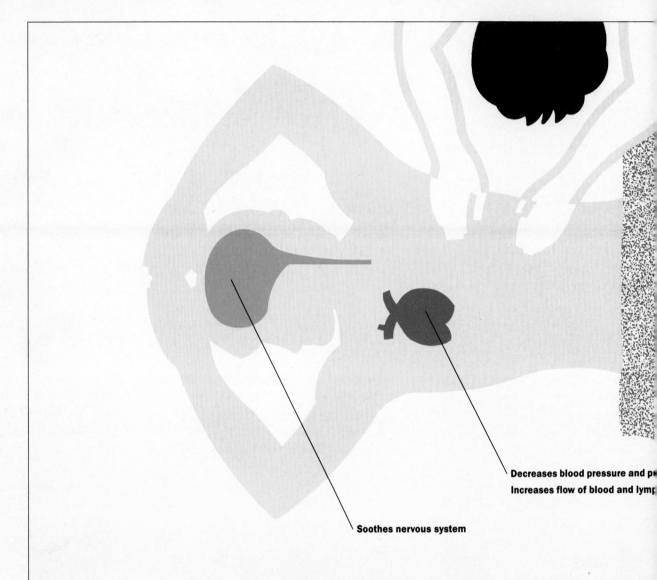

Decreases blood pressure and p◼

Increases flow of blood and lym◼

Soothes nervous system

How Massage Benefits the Body

Massage does more than make you feel good — it has wide-ranging physiological effects. Its initial benefits stem from the stimulation of nerve receptors in the skin. The nerve impulses, triggered by rhythmic massage motions, are relayed to the central nervous system (the brain and spinal cord), where they are translated into messages of relaxation that are sent back to the muscles. One type of massage stroke, the nerve stroke, calms and soothes peripheral nerve endings in the skin.

Massage has an effect on the circulatory system. Studies have shown that various massage strokes cause capillaries beneath the skin to expand, thus increasing the flow of blood. Since many strokes are done in a centripetal direction — toward the heart — they speed the flow of deoxygenated blood from muscle cells to the heart and lungs, where the blood is replenished with oxygen.

Furthermore, the increase in blood flow due to massage can produce a temporary decrease in blood

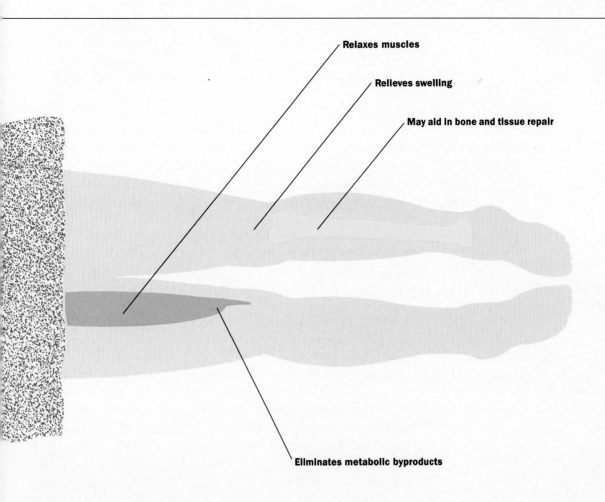

Relaxes muscles

Relieves swelling

May aid in bone and tissue repair

Eliminates metabolic byproducts

pressure. Researchers have found that massage also slows the pulse rate and promotes relaxed breathing, two indicators of reduced stress.

Massage also encourages the flow of lymph, a colorless fluid that transports proteins and other substances from the muscles and bones to the blood. The increased lymph flow helps prevent fluid accumulation that can lead to swollen tissues and joints.

The muscular system can benefit from massage in several ways. First, massage stretches and relaxes muscles, promotes flexibility and increases the range of motion. Massage also helps tired or injured muscles recuperate by mechanically ridding them of lactic acid, a metabolic by-product *(see page 11)*.

Some evidence suggests that massage affects the skeletal system. In one experiment, massaging the area around fractured bones significantly increased the retention of nitrogen, sulfur and phosphorus, all of which are necessary for repair of injured tissue.

What is massage?

Massage is the systematic manipulation of the body's soft tissues, primarily the muscles, to benefit the nervous, muscular and circulatory systems. Usually this manipulation is performed with the hands, although some forms of massage also use the forearms, elbows, knees and even the feet.

Massage may be the oldest method of treating human ills. It is mentioned in a Chinese medical tract dating back 3,000 years and in the annals of ancient Egypt, Greece and Rome. Massage probably originated from our natural impulse to rub an ache or a bump to relieve pain. Over time this "rubbing" has been formalized into a number of different movements applied to specific parts of the body. Most forms of massage involve combinations of these movements, which include stroking, kneading, wringing, pulling, vibrating, percussing (tapping or striking) and pressing. Each of these is shown in detail in Chapter Two.

Are there different schools of massage?

Massage has become an umbrella term for many methods of body manipulation. Most of these can be grouped into two basic schools. The Western school, the so-called structure-based system, arises from a European tradition that focuses on the body's musculoskeletal system. The most widely used Western method is Swedish massage, originally designed to duplicate the muscle movements of Swedish gymnastics through body manipulation.

Eastern forms of massage are "energy-based" systems derived from the theory that a vital force circulates throughout the body. When this force is blocked by tension or injury, illness or pain results. The aim of Eastern techniques is to unblock areas where this force has become trapped, thus restoring the flow of energy. The best-known Eastern school is shiatsu, which uses pressure on various vital points called *tsubos* to free blocked energy. Acupressure and reflexology, which also involve applying pressure at vital points, are among the other energy-based types of massage.

Sports massage is a relatively new type of massage that combines the strokes of Swedish massage with the pressure-point techniques of Eastern massage. Much of the current interest in massage in general stems from the acceptance of sports massage as a regular part of training by a growing number of professional athletes. Unlike other forms of massage, sports massage focuses on specific muscles or muscle groups. Furthermore, it is used not only to maintain healthy muscles, but also to rehabilitate injured tissue.

Is one type of massage more effective than another?

Increasingly, the line between Eastern and Western methods is being blurred: Massage therapists have realized that these techniques are not mutually exclusive, but in fact can complement each other. Some of the whole-body strokes of Swedish massage, for example, also affect

Massage and Muscle Recovery

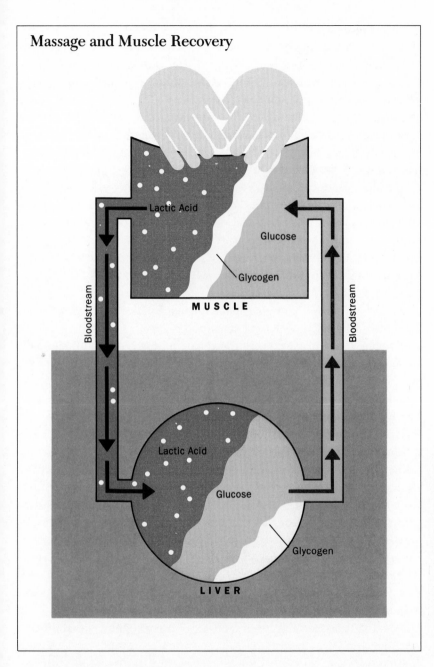

During exercise, glucose and oxygen are delivered to the muscles and converted into glycogen, a source of energy for them. When exercise is long or strenuous, this process becomes less efficient and allows the build-up of lactic acid, a by-product of energy production that tires the muscles and may cause soreness. By "milking" the muscles, massage speeds the removal of lactic acid, which is carried through the bloodstream to the liver and resynthesized into glucose. The glucose is then converted into glycogen in the liver and muscles. One study showed that muscles sore from exercise recovered their efficiency more quickly with massage than with a rest period alone.

a number of the pressure points of shiatsu, and many massage therapists now use the two disciplines in tandem. Therefore, in this book, one chapter shows you how to give a whole-body massage that incorporates Swedish techniques with those of shiatsu and reflexology. Another chapter, on sports massage, focuses on individual muscle groups and injury prevention.

What are the principal effects of massage?

First and foremost, the rhythmic movements of massage induce relaxation, which prepares the muscles for several other direct physiological changes, known as mechanical effects. Most significant, massage enlarges blood vessels, thereby increasing circulation. Because most strokes are performed in the direction of the heart — from the foot to the thigh, for example — they speed the passage of deoxygenated blood back to the heart, where it is replenished with oxygen and returned to the muscles to help supply them with energy. By the same process, massage also quickens the removal from the muscles of lactic acid, a by-product of muscular activity that causes fatigue.

Is a back rub just as effective?
No, although there is evidence that part of the effectiveness of massage stems from the simple act of touching. To this extent, a back rub can help you relax and may even soothe minor, local aches, but the more comprehensive effects of massage are the result of rigorous and systematic routines, such as those demonstrated in this book, that benefit your circulatory, muscular and nervous systems.

Can massage relieve stress-related problems like headaches?
Because of its soothing effect on muscles, massage can help relieve headaches that are caused by muscular tension, usually in the face, neck and upper back. Such tension, in fact, is a common response to stress, so it follows that massage works well to reduce stress. Besides promoting relaxation, some types of massage can temporarily lower the heart and pulse rates, two further signs of stress reduction, and can contribute to slower, more relaxed respiration.

Moreover, massage can elevate mood and promote a sense of well-being. In one study, researchers undertook a massage program with anxious patients who did not respond well to drug therapy and had difficulty relaxing. After a series of at least 10 massage sessions lasting 30 to 45 minutes apiece, all the patients said they felt more relaxed, were experiencing fewer distress symptoms and were sleeping better. Some of them discontinued their drugs and others were able to get along with lower dosages.

Can you treat more serious conditions with massage?
Claims that massage has been successful in curing chronic illness are not supported by scientific evidence. Research has shown, however, that massage can decrease high blood pressure, although this effect is usually short-lived. Some physicians also prescribe back and chest massage to loosen bronchial secretions in patients with asthma and chronic bronchitis. And there are indications that massaging premature infants can promote their growth and muscle function.

There is also some evidence that because of its ability to increase blood flow, massage may aid in bone and tissue repair, and many physical therapists include massage in their treatment of fractures. One study showed that massaging the area around a broken limb substantially increased the retention of nitrogen, sulfur and phosphorus, all of which are necessary for tissue repair.

Many researchers believe that part of the efficacy of massage lies simply in the healing power of touch. In one study, a nurse persuaded 32 of her colleagues to use touching — placing a hand on someone's shoulder, for example — when caring for hospitalized patients. All of the patients who had been touched showed significant increases in their level of hemoglobin, a substance in red blood cells that carries oxygen to the tissues.

The Flexibility Factor

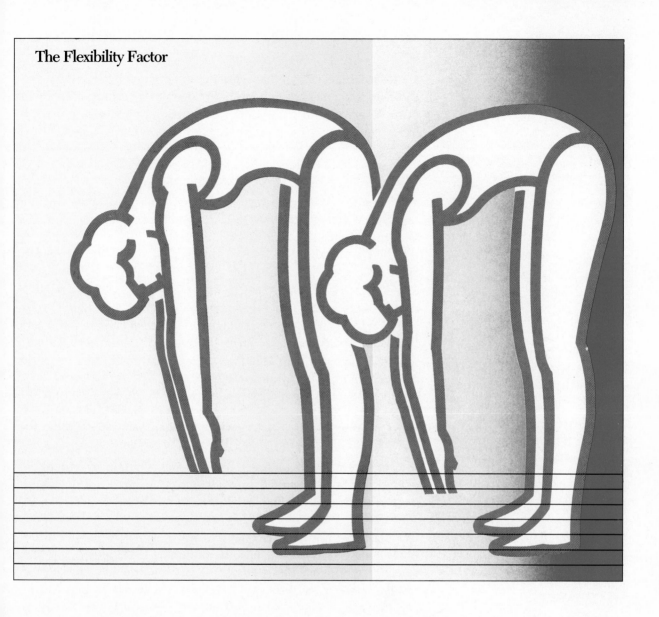

Is massage a good remedy for back pain?

Massage can help back and other musculoskeletal pain by breaking the so-called pain cycle — a mechanism whereby the initial cause of pain triggers muscle spasms that impair circulation and in turn produce more pain. By relaxing muscles and restoring circulation, massage can interrupt this cycle and thus relieve the pain. Some researchers also believe that manual manipulation of the skin and underlying tissues prompts a release of certain chemicals in the body that reduce pain and anxiety. Researchers theorize that this phenomenon may partly explain the effectiveness of both shiatsu and acupressure, which relieve pain by manipulating the same pressure points that acupuncture reaches with needles.

The principal effect of massage is to loosen and relax taut muscles, which can significantly enhance flexibility. In one study, 25 subjects were asked to touch their toes, a flexibility test for the back, hips, buttocks and back of the legs. They were then given a 30-minute back and hip massage, after which they repeated the test. Each of the subjects could reach farther after the massage than before. The mean gain was 1.35 inches, as the two figures above indicate.

Cross-Fiber Massage

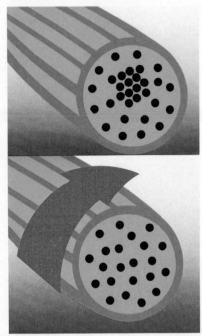

Muscles function by alternately contracting and relaxing. But injury or overuse can cause the individual fibers within a muscle to stick together, limiting their contraction *(top)*. Cross-fiber, or deep-friction, massage, which is applied across the grain of the muscle fibers, as the arrow indicates *(above)*, can separate matted fibers. Used regularly, cross-fiber massage helps to prevent injury and keep muscles functioning optimally.

Do doctors often prescribe massage?

Over the past few years, massage has won wider acceptance among physicians, especially in the treatment of neck and back problems. In addition, some massage schools have begun to specialize in therapeutic massage, and many leading health insurers now cover massage treatments if a doctor prescribes them. The growing acceptance of massage by the medical profession has perhaps been spurred by the burgeoning field of sports medicine, where massage has come to play a vital role. Many professional athletes — and their team physicians — now consider regular massage an indispensable part of the training regimen. When combined with rest, sports massage can enable athletes to recover more quickly after a workout.

How do athletes use massage?

Sports massage is a four-part regimen designed to aid the athlete in training, both before and after a competition or workout, and in rehabilitation from injury. The techniques used at each of these times vary. Preventive sports massage, which is demonstrated in this volume, is used in training to help keep the exerciser injury-free, and so allow him or her to work to maximum capacity. The pre-event massage stimulates circulation and promotes muscle flexibility, both of which help prepare the muscles for the upcoming activity and reduce the risk of injury. After exercise, the task of massage is not to stimulate and prepare muscles, but to relax them and aid in their recovery. Rehabilitative sports massage benefits the recently or chronically injured athlete. Because it involves diagnosis and work on injured tissue, this type of massage is best left to a licensed professional.

Can massage improve performance during exercise or competition?

Many athletes and trainers have reported that massage boosts performance. Experiments designed to test this have yielded contradictory results, however. In one study, massage was shown to improve the performance of male and female athletes in a series of swimming, running and cycling events. Other researchers have found no such effect, but massage therapists point out that many benefits of massage are cumulative and are not as pronounced after a single massage. Based on the available clinical evidence, though, it seems clear that massage can enhance performance in at least one respect: Flexible, relaxed muscles are better able to withstand the rigors of strenuous exercise, and muscles that recover quickly from exertion can engage in more frequent bouts of training.

Can massage condition muscles as effectively as exercise?

No. Although massage can help prepare muscles for exertion and reduce the likelihood of injury, a muscle's strength, size and endurance must be built with exercise that makes it work. To increase flexibility substantially, you need to use massage in conjunction with a program of stretching exercises.

Will massage help you lose weight?

Some enthusiasts have claimed that massage can break down fat deposits beneath the skin, and massage is often used in combination with steam-bath treatments at weight-reducing salons. But any weight lost by such a regimen is water, which you will quickly regain. You can keep weight off only by exercising and by dieting properly.

How effective is self-massage?

If a massage partner is not available, self-massage is an acceptable alternative for reducing stress-induced tension and for soothing over-exerted muscles. But self-massage has two inherent limitations. First, there are a number of important muscles — those of the upper back, for example — that you cannot effectively massage on your own. Second, the very nature of putting forth an effort yourself during massage defeats one of its major purposes, relaxation, which presumes that the person receiving the massage be inactive.

How long should a massage treatment last?

There is no set time limit. Deep-friction or cross-fiber sports massage, which works a particular muscle group deeply and specifically, will usually last no more than 10 minutes. A relaxing full-body massage, on the other hand, might require a full hour. For more details on the length of the various massage routines presented in this volume, see the chart on page 21.

Are there times when you should not receive a massage?

If you have a serious or chronic illness, it is best to check with your doctor before getting a massage. Generally speaking, experts advise against massage when you have a fever or any type of infection, since a massage could aggravate its spread through your body. Similarly, you should not have a massage if you are suffering from phlebitis, tumors, thrombosis or varicose veins, as massage may dislodge blood clots associated with these conditions. Also avoid massage if you have any skin eruptions, like poison ivy, that are contagious or could be spread by contact. Likewise, you should not give a massage if you have an infectious illness or sores on your hands. Pregnant women should avoid abdominal message.

How should you use this book?

The following chapters illustrate basic techniques for giving a thorough massage. Bear in mind that only a licensed massage therapist is trained to use massage for treating injuries; if you suspect you have an injury, you should consult your physician before receiving a massage. But you can learn to give a massage that is designed to relax your partner or, in the case of sports massage, help prevent fatigue and injury to specific muscles. The next few pages will help you decide which massage techniques are best suited for you and your partner.

How to Design Your Own Program

You can use massage in a variety of ways, from reducing day-to-day stress to relieving soreness or preventing injury in specific muscles. The remaining pages in this chapter will help you assess how you and your partner might like to take advantage of massage and guide you to the proper techniques.

How relaxed are you?

1 **Do you have a high-stress job?**

Work-related pressures are a major contributor to stress, which can first manifest itself as muscular tension. One of the primary and immediate benefits of massage is relaxation. In fact, the stress-reducing benefits of massage have proven so effective that a growing number of companies are incorporating massage into their fitness programs; some have even made in-office massage available to their employees. If you do feel stress building up during the day, you can help alleviate it with the office massage presented on pages 24-27.

2 **Do you frequently feel tired?**

Massage can relieve both muscular and mental fatigue. By improving your circulation, massage speeds the replacement of deoxygenated blood with oxygen-rich blood to the muscles. It will also help cleanse the muscles of lactic acid, which many researchers believe contributes to muscle fatigue and soreness. Because lactic acid and other metabolic by-products are released into the bloodstream during a massage, you may still feel tired immediately afterward. But this effect is only temporary. These substances are carried to the heart or liver, where they are either eliminated or remetabolized; as this occurs, your energy level will rise. Also, certain massage strokes are specifically designed to soothe nerves.

3 **How often is a massage necessary to keep muscles relaxed?**

No studies have established how the frequency of massage affects the benefits to your body. But, based on the clinical experience of massage therapists, the effects of massage are cumulative, so that regular sessions at least once a week can promote long-lasting muscle relaxation and a general reduction in fatigue.

4 **Do you suffer from back pain?**

Increasingly, doctors, osteopaths and chiropractors are recommending massage, usually in conjunction with physical therapy, to help relieve back pain. With any back pain, you should first consult a doctor. But if you are not suffering from a debilitating injury, you can use massage to ease muscle soreness and tension in your back.

5 Does your face show signs of tension?

A knitted brow, clenched jaw and tight lips are all signs of emotion-related muscular tension. Indeed, studies have shown that the face is one of the primary areas in the body in which tension occurs and is most evident. You can reduce this tension with cosmetic massage, using strokes such as those shown on pages 90-93. Cosmetic massage cannot erase wrinkles — only plastic surgery can do that. But it can relax and tone the many muscles of the face, improve circulation to the skin and help ease stress-related headaches.

6 What kind of exercise do you do?

Different exercises place stress on different muscles. And many exercises place uneven stress on your musculoskeletal system: Tennis, for example, can lead to more muscle development in one arm and on one side of your neck than the other. Overtraining and general wear and tear can affect any exercise participant, leading to soreness, fatigue and sometimes injury.

You can help keep your muscles in optimal condition with sports massage, which works on specific muscles to lengthen and separate muscle fibers, thereby reducing soreness, tightness and the likelihood of injury. In addition, there is a growing body of clinical evidence that sports massage can aid your performance and improve your recovery time after a workout. To see which massage strokes are best suited to your particular exercise, see pages 22-23.

7 If you have never given a massage, what is the best way to start?

Since you are working with another person's body, it is understandable if you feel somewhat nervous at first. Your relationship with your massage partner is very important, and one way to gain trust in one another is to receive as well as give a massage. Not only will this put you and your partner on an equal footing, but it will allow you to better experience and assess the various massage techniques. This book, therefore, is really intended to be shared.

In addition, you may feel more comfortable with certain strokes or styles of massage — for example, you may first prefer to try reflexology, in which you need only remove your shoes, or shiatsu, during which you can wear loose-fitting clothing. These and other options are presented in the following pages, so respect your partner's wishes — the more relaxed about the experience he or she is, the more effective and enjoyable the massage will be.

Easing Tense Muscles

Certain areas of your body are vulnerable to muscle soreness from everyday stresses. A high-pressured, sedentary job, or any situation that causes you to maintain a rigid position for hours at a time, can result in your muscles shortening, which may produce discomfort. One of the prime advantages of massage is that it eases such tension-related aches.

Many people, for example, find that they experience a great deal of tension in the numerous small muscles of the face and neck — a "tension triangle" with its base at the top of the shoulders and its apex in the forehead. In fact, the muscles of the brow — the corrugator muscles — are considered such an accurate gauge of tension throughout the body that they are used in biofeedback training to monitor stress. In one study, researchers found that subjects who were depressed had chronically tensed corrugators, even when they did not appear to be frowning or knitting their brows.

Among the most uncomfortable on-the-job muscular aches — and the most common — are those affecting the trapezius, the large triangular muscle that extends downward from the neck to the shoulder blades. This muscle helps hold up the head, which weighs an average of 10 pounds. Leaning forward over a desk for long periods strains the trapezius, as does cradling a telephone between your ear and shoulder.

Work-related tension can manifest itself in the shoulders, arms and hands, particularly if you use a computer keyboard or a typewriter. If you sit a great deal, the strain may show up in your lower back. Being sedentary can also generate muscular tension in your legs, although a more likely cause of sore leg muscles is overexertion during exercise or sports (see pages 22-23). In addition, your abdomen can become tense, especially if you unconsciously tend to hold your breath during moments of emotional stress or concentration.

Use the illustration opposite to pinpoint your particular tight spots and the massage techniques that can alleviate them.

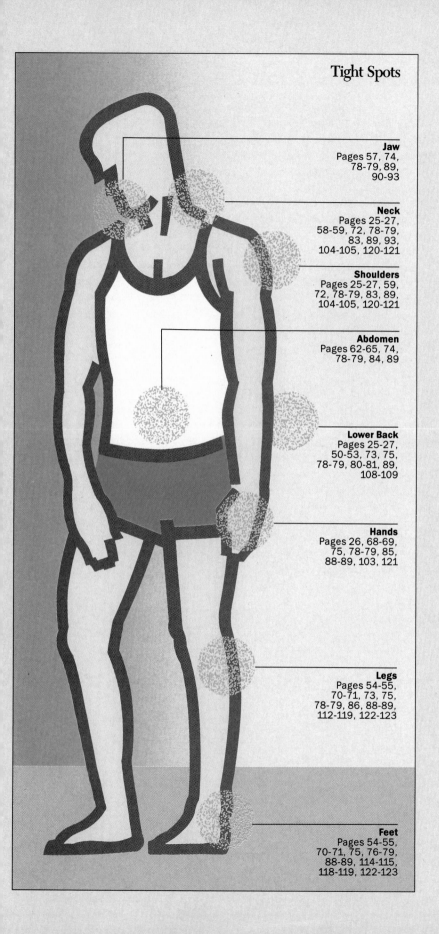

Tight Spots

Jaw
Pages 57, 74,
78-79, 89,
90-93

Neck
Pages 25-27,
58-59, 72, 78-79,
83, 89, 93,
104-105, 120-121

Shoulders
Pages 25-27, 59,
72, 78-79, 83, 89,
104-105, 120-121

Abdomen
Pages 62-65, 74,
78-79, 84, 89

Lower Back
Pages 25-27,
50-53, 73, 75,
78-79, 80-81, 89,
108-109

Hands
Pages 26, 68-69,
75, 78-79, 85,
88-89, 103, 121

Legs
Pages 54-55,
70-71, 73, 75,
78-79, 86, 88-89,
112-119, 122-123

Feet
Pages 54-55,
70-71, 75, 76-79,
88-89, 114-115,
118-119, 122-123

Choosing Your Massage

Massage gives you many options, from a relaxing full-body session to an intense sports massage. Within this broad spectrum, you can select a traditional, Swedish-based head-to-toe massage or choose shiatsu, an Oriental full-body routine. If you are pressed for time, you might choose a quick upper body massage or a five-minute reflexology tune-up; if you have just finished a workout but have no available partner, you may benefit from sports self-massage.

As the chart opposite shows, you can adapt massage to your schedule, your location and the equipment at hand. And if your situation — or your partner — changes, you can select another type of massage that is more appropriate. Just remember that the most important criterion for choosing a massage is that it be comfortable for you to give as well as for your partner to receive.

A Massage Guide

Type	Benefits	Time Required	Equipment	Pages
FULL-BODY	Incorporating the most familiar Swedish-based techniques, full-body massage relaxes the entire body. It benefits the nervous, circulatory and musculoskeletal systems, and promotes a general sense of psychological well-being.	From 45 minutes to an hour	A well-padded floor or a massage table; oil; pillows to place under neck and knees (optional); towels, sheets or blankets for draping.	32-41, 50-71
SHIATSU	According to Oriental precepts, shiatsu will balance your body's energy to produce an invigorated feeling. You need to learn only one simple pressure technique. Your partner can wear a leotard or loose-fitting clothes; a massage table is unnecessary; oil is not used.	From 20 to 30 minutes	None	45, 72-75
REFLEXOLOGY	Because you need only to remove your partner's shoes and socks, reflexology can be done almost anytime or anywhere. In theory, you can treat the entire body just by pressing various points on the feet. You can also perform reflexology on yourself.	Working on a specific body part or area can take five minutes; a full treatment takes about 30 minutes.	Oil or lotion is optional; a reclining chair or massage table can be used if desired.	76-79, 88-89
SPORTS	Sports massage works specific muscle groups used in exercise to increase muscular flexibility and reduce the likelihood of injury. Some evidence suggests a possible connection with improved athletic performance.	From 15 to 30 minutes	A massage table is best, but you can also use the floor. Towels and sheets for draping are used, as is oil.	40-45, 98-119
COSMETIC	Cosmetic massage treats the face, head and neck to increase circulation to the skin and enhance muscular flexibility; this improves skin tone and appearance.	15 minutes	Moisturizing facial lotion.	90-93
SELF-MASSAGE/ FULL BODY	The advantage of self-massage is that you do not need a partner. It can ease some degree of muscular tension and relax you. It also provides an opportunity to practice your techniques.	About 20 minutes	Oil	32-39, 45, 80-87
SELF-MASSAGE/ SPORTS	A primary advantage of sports self-massage is that it is immediately available, even if you are in the midst of exercising. It is particularly effective on the lower body, where you can get the most leverage.	From five to 20 minutes	None	40-45, 120-123
QUICK MASSAGE	Quick massage can relieve common neck, shoulder and back tension. Since your partner can remain seated and fully clothed, this routine can even be done in an office.	10 minutes	None	24-27

Improving Your Game

The various sports you play affect the muscles in your body differently. Even when two activities involve the same body parts, the specific muscles that are engaged will differ. Although running and tennis both use the leg, for example, they focus on separate sets of leg muscles.

Such differences are the basis for sports massage: It is sports-specific, concentrating on the particular muscles most used in an activity, rather than on the whole body. So a cyclist and a runner will receive different massages, as will a basketball player and a baseball player.

The chart opposite pairs common sports and fitness activities with the appropriate preventive sports-massage techniques you should use to keep your muscles flexible, enabling you to recover sooner from postexercise soreness.

Included in the chart are injuries associated with the various sports to help you pinpoint potential trouble spots. Evidence suggests that preventive sports massage may reduce the likelihood of injury; however, if you suspect that you have any of these conditions, seek advice from your physician. Sudden, severe or chronic pain should be diagnosed before you embark on a massage program, and any rehabilitative massage prescribed should be performed only by a licensed therapist.

AEROBIC DANCE
pages 108-109, 112-119

While this activity works your whole body, improper landing places a great deal of stress on the lower body. The most common complaints mimic those of runners: shin splints, knee strain, foot pain, calf pulls and lower back strain.

BASEBALL/SOFTBALL
pages 98-107

Postworkout soreness in these activities tends to result from insufficient conditioning; it occurs mainly in the shoulder, arm, chest and upper back muscles, which are used for throwing.

BASKETBALL
pages 98-105, 112-119

The stop-and-go action of basketball stresses the leg, especially the ankle, knee and hip joints; the chest, arms and shoulders are used for dribbling and shooting. Possible injuries include sprained ankles, knee strain, and hip and hamstring pulls.

CYCLING
pages 100-105, 108-109, 112-119

Like running, cycling mostly stresses the legs, but it also causes tension in the hands, lower back, neck and shoulders. Common cyclists' complaints are knee and wrist strain, as well as tight quadriceps.

FOOTBALL
pages 104-105, 108-109, 112-113, 116-117

Because it is a contact sport, football can injure almost any muscle in the body. Particularly vulnerable muscles are those in the neck, shoulder, lower back and thighs.

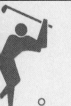

GOLF
pages 98-109

Although golf is not considered a strenuous sport, frequent bending can strain the lower back. Golf also requires fine muscle coordination and shoulder flexibility, which can be aided mainly by massage to the arms, chest and back.

RACQUET SPORTS
pages 100-105, 112-119

Tennis, racquetball and squash all place uneven stress on the arms, shoulders and neck, so these are the primary areas to concentrate on during massage. Massage can also help the leg muscles, which are subjected to rapid stop-and-go action in these sports.

ROWING
pages 100-109, 116-117

Rowing relies on both upper arm and leg strength, and uses the back extensively; yet it has a low injury rate. You will benefit especially from massage to the arms, quadriceps and back.

RUNNING/WALKING
pages 110-119

These sports primarily use the leg muscles, especially the calf muscles and the hamstrings. Massaging the legs will help you to avoid the most common injuries, including Achilles tendinitis, strained gluteals, heel pain, shin splints and pulled hamstrings.

SKIING
pages 100-105, 108-109, 114-119

Downhill and cross-country skiers are prone to stress in the lower back, quadriceps and calves. Strenuous poling in cross-country skiing may also strain the arms and shoulders.

SOCCER
pages 110-119

The leg muscles are used extensively for both speed and endurance in soccer. Rapid stopping and starting can injure the knees and pull thigh muscles. Also, repeated kicking can fully extend—and strain—the gluteals.

SWIMMING
pages 100-107

This sport, which benefits nearly all of the body's major muscle groups, is less likely to cause injury than weight-bearing exercises. However, possible trouble spots are the arms, shoulders and neck.

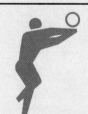

VOLLEYBALL
pages 100-105, 112-119

Volleyball makes extensive use of the hands, arms and shoulders. It also relies on jumping, which can strain the leg joints.

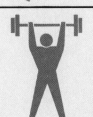

WEIGHT LIFTING
pages 98-99, 104-105, 108-109, 116-119

Most weight lifters try to build their entire body, alternating upper and lower body workouts. Shoulder and lower back strains are common problems, but the chest and knees also merit massage.

Quick Massage/1

To be effective, a thorough full-body massage requires a table or floor, oil and a minimum of 45 minutes. But you can reduce a good deal of the tension and stress that build up during the day with the massage routine shown on the following three pages, which takes only 15 minutes.

While the goal of most massage is relaxation, this routine is energizing. It was originally created as an on-the-job massage for office workers, but because it requires little time and no equipment, this invigorating treatment can be given anytime and anywhere. Designed to be performed while your partner is sitting and fully clothed, the routine does not require any oil. All of the strokes are targeted at those areas of the upper body — particularly the trapezius muscle running down the neck and upper back and the erector spinae muscles running along either side of the back — where work-related muscular tension frequently occurs. You will also do some strokes on the arms and hands, which are integrally involved in most daily work.

The strokes of quick massage are modifications of traditional massage; to execute them properly, you should first familiarize yourself with the basic techniques shown in the next chapter.

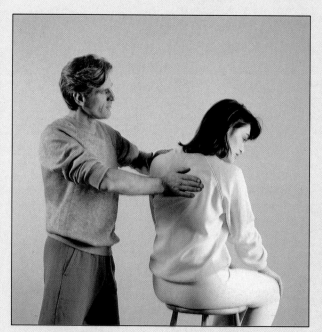

Cup your left hand around your partner's left shoulder and place your right palm on the left side of her spine. Start at the top of her back and press next to her spine. Repeat five times, working downward to just above her waist; switch sides.

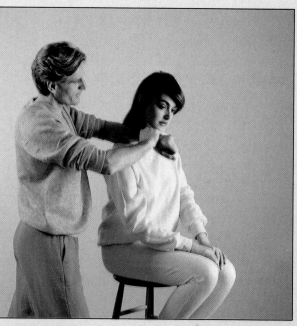

Grasp your left wrist with your right hand. Place your forearm at the base of the right side of your partner's neck. Press down with your forearm. Move toward the shoulder, pressing two more times at three-quarter-inch intervals. Repeat the sequence; switch sides.

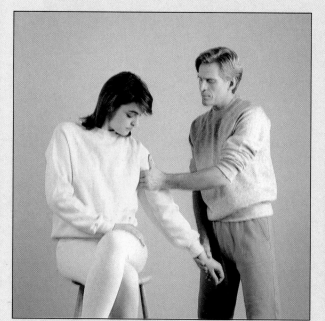

With one hand, hold your partner's arm away from her body and grasp the inside of her upper arm with the other hand. With your thumb perpendicular to her shoulder, squeeze her biceps at five equidistant points down to her elbow. Perform five times.

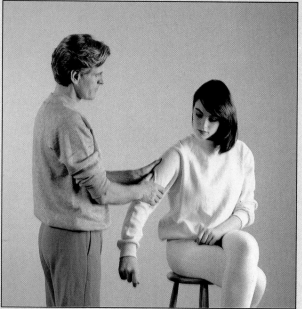

Grasp your partner's arm near her shoulder, with your left thumb perpendicular to the shoulder. Press, then place your right thumb beneath the left and press again. Continue alternating pressure to work down the arm to above the elbow. Perform five times.

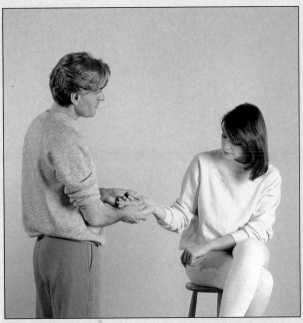

Turn your partner's hand palm up. Cover her palm with small circular movements of your thumb. Then grasp her thumb between your thumb and forefinger. Alternately rub your fingers back and forth, working toward the tip. Repeat on each of her fingers.

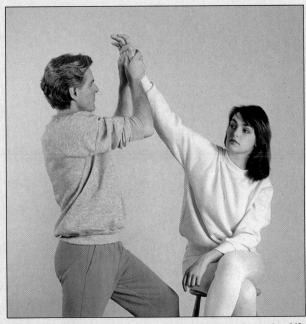

Hold your partner's hand so that your thumbs grasp her palm. Lift her arm up and away from her body, as if she were reaching to pick an apple. This will loosen the muscles of her shoulder joint. Repeat this stroke and the three previous strokes on her other arm.

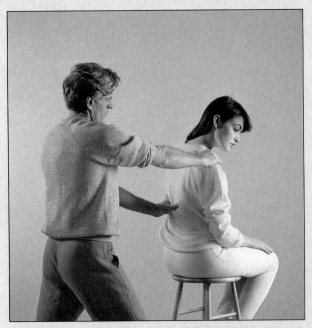

Cup your right hand over your partner's right shoulder as a brace. Use your left thumb to press deeply into the muscle running along the right side of her spine. Start just below her shoulder blade and work down to her waist; repeat on the other side.

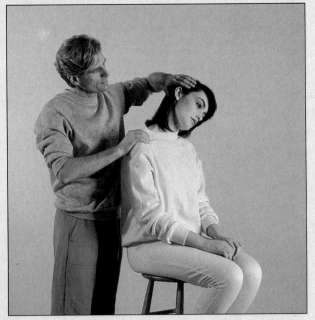

Again, cup your right hand over your partner's right shoulder as a brace. Cup your other hand over her right ear. Simultaneously press down on her shoulder and gently push her head to the left. Repeat twice, then switch sides.

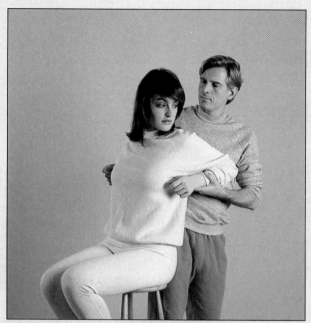

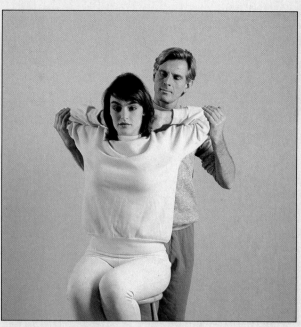

Bend both of your partner's arms at the elbow. Place your hip against her lower back as a brace and grasp both her forearms just below the elbow. Gently pull her arms up and straight back. Repeat twice. This will stretch her entire upper back.

Have your partner interlock her hands behind her neck. Again, place your hip against her lower back as a brace. As she exhales, pull her elbows slightly back. Perform three times to work her chest and shoulder muscles.

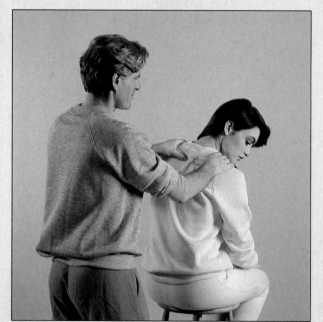

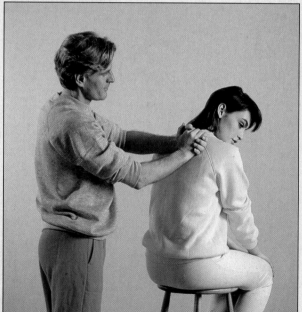

Grasp the base of your partner's neck with both hands. Do four semicircular rotations with your thumbs, working out toward her shoulders. Bring your hands back toward her neck with four more rotations, then do four rotations downward next to the spine.

Cup your hands loosely. Bend your wrists and tap your partner's back lightly and rapidly. Start at the left shoulder and tap toward the neck, then down the left side of the spine, up the right side and across the right side of the shoulder. Avoid the spine itself.

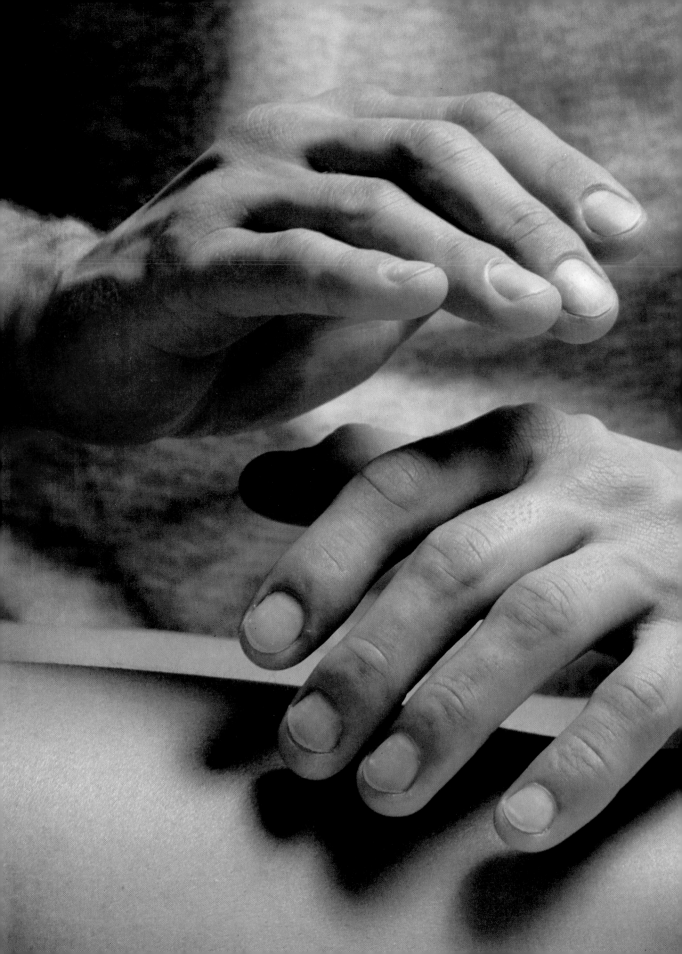

CHAPTER TWO

Basic Techniques

Becoming proficient at massage: the right strokes and their effects

To give a massage that is both relaxing and therapeutic, you need to learn five basic hand movements: stroking, compression, percussion, friction and pressure. Each movement, derived from an Eastern or Western massage discipline, has a specific physiological effect that you can control by the way you perform it — for example, whether you stroke on the surface of the skin or deeply into muscle tissue.

Probably the most basic and well-known massage stroke is effleurage (French for "stroke" or "glide"). When done lightly, as in the nerve stroke *(page 33)*, effleurage is relaxing. When performed more forcefully, as in the deep stroke associated with sports massage *(page 43)*, it enhances drainage of the lymph system and promotes better circulation by opening blood vessels and capillaries.

Compression techniques, which include petrissage (French for "knead") and sports-massage compressions, are shown on pages 34-35 and page 44. The effect of these techniques is to move muscle away from or across bone, which improves oxygenation of the muscle, removes metabolic by-products and increases circulation.

Friction and both broad and local cross-fiber stroking *(pages 36-37 and page 42)* are movements that work deeply into a joint or muscle to increase flexibility and mobility. Percussive techniques *(pages 38-39)* require gentle striking of a specific area. Because this type of movement contracts your muscles and increases their blood supply, it can feel stimulating. But when sustained for more than 10 seconds, it has a relaxing effect. Vibration and jostling *(pages 40-41)*, although not percussive movements, produce similar results: Vibration can be either stimulating or sedating, and jostling is soothing.

Pressure movements *(page 45)* are the mainstay of Eastern massage therapies like shiatsu and reflexology. And they are used in Western massage — and sports massage in particular — on trigger points, localized spots in muscles where crystallized metabolic by-products reduce blood supply and cause pain. Pressure movements are applied to a specific site with the thumb or fingers.

Through practice, you will learn just how deeply to work when performing a particular technique. Generally, you can apply more pressure to fleshy parts of the body like the thighs and buttocks. Direct pressure is never used on bones, so work around such areas as the knees, elbows and shoulder blades. Likewise, because of potential danger to the vertebrae, never put any pressure on the spine.

When massaging a particular area, look for a flush or redness there. This is called hyperemia, and it occurs when blood rises to the skin's surface due to the increase in circulation that an effective massage produces. While hyperemia is expected and encouraged, you should never massage so strenuously that swelling results.

For the most part, a massage should not cause pain. However, some of the techniques mentioned above can occasionally produce discomfort, depending on where and how they are performed. In fact, pain is an integral part of some pressure techniques. When you press a trigger point, for example, your massage partner may initially feel pain, but this sensation should subside within a few seconds, as the pressure releases the accumulated metabolic by-products. The amount of discomfort allowed should be determined by your partner's pain threshold, as well as his or her present physical condition. If you are working on a sore area, for example, you might need to decrease the force you would normally use. It is a good practice to ask your partner how he or she is feeling throughout the massage. These responses, coupled with his or her body signals — a sudden jerk, say, or a tensed muscle — will enable you to determine where to exert pressure and how much.

In most instances, you should massage toward the heart to aid the flow of venous, or deoxygenated, blood and lymph. Use smooth and rhythmic movements to maximize the effectiveness of the massage and your partner's comfort. Keep both hands in contact with your partner, even when only one hand is stroking. This 10-point touch, as

Tools for Massage

◆ You can give a massage on a massage table or on the floor. A table is preferable because it allows you to move around easily and does not strain your knees or back, as kneeling on the floor can. Massage tables are available in wood and aluminum, and measure about six feet by two feet. Adjust the table to the height of the top of your thighs. Place a one-inch-thick foam pad on top; before giving a massage, cover the pad with a clean sheet to protect it from oil.

◆ If you perform a massage on the floor, pad the surface with a one- to two-inch-thick piece of foam that measures about seven feet by four feet. (This allows you room to kneel on the padding.) You can also use an exercise mat or layers of blankets. Cover these surfaces with a sheet.

◆ You should use oil for all the massage techniques presented on the following pages except the friction and pressure work on pages 36-37 and page 45. Oil allows your hands to glide over your partner's body, prevents rubbing and reduces pulling on body hair. You can purchase prepared massage oils at many health stores, but ordinary vegetable and mineral oils are also fine and usually less expensive. Sesame, peanut and almond oils are among those favored by massage therapists. Keep the oil in a plastic, not a glass, container to avoid accidental breakage; it should be at room temperature or slightly warmer. Pour oil onto your hands and then use effleurage, shown on the next page, to spread it. Apply only a thin film on your partner's body — about half a teaspoon is sufficient for most areas.

massage therapists call it, alleviates any apprehension your partner may feel about what either hand is going to do next.

Position yourself so that you can perform a stroke with minimal movement by either you or your partner. Massage symmetrically, working both sides of the body equally and with the same techniques. And synchronize your breathing with your partner's — both of you exhaling as you stroke outward and inhaling as you glide back — to maximize the effectiveness of the stroke.

Draping your partner properly is also important. Not only does it respect your partner's modesty, but it also keeps him or her warm. While the increased blood flow will warm the area being massaged, the rest of your partner's body, which is in a relaxed, almost sleeplike, state, can become chilled. Therefore, expose only the area you are working on. *(For instructions on draping, see page 49.)* In addition, your hands should be warm, as should any lotion or oil you intend to use *(see box above)*. Keep your fingernails closely clipped.

The following pages will teach you the basic techniques of massage. (For visual clarity, most of the strokes are demonstrated on the back.) Chapters Three and Four will develop these techniques into sequences for Swedish massage, sports massage and other types. Take time both to practice and experience the techniques with your partner. Knowing how the stroke feels on you will help you give a better massage, and communicating during massage — ideally with comments only on the massage process — will increase your skill.

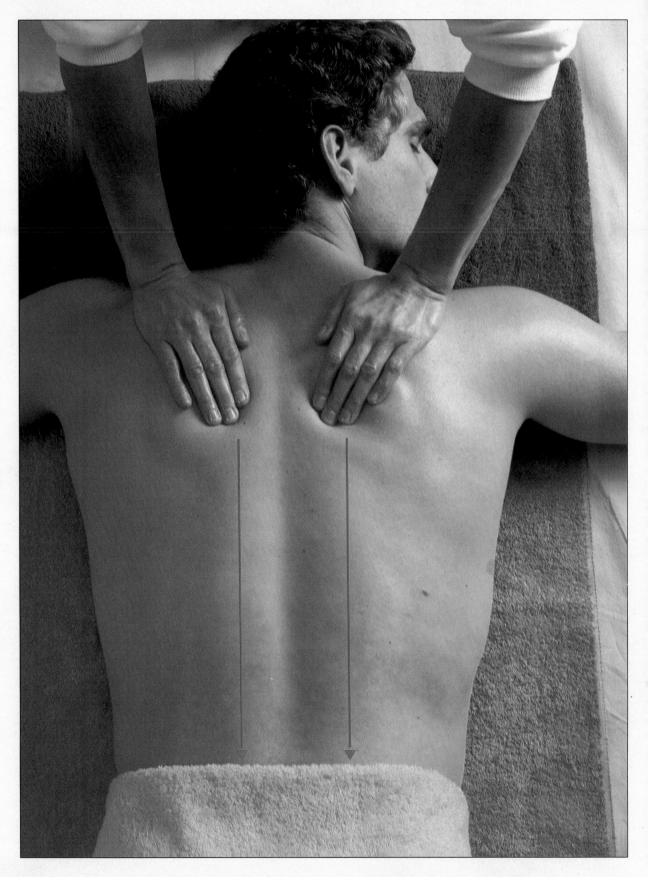

Effleurage

Most massages begin and end with effleurage, a slow, rhythmic stroke that is performed with your fingertips, palms, thumbs or knuckles, depending on how deeply you want to work the muscles. Generally, effleurage works from the extremities toward the heart — from the wrist to the shoulder, for example. An exception is the nerve stroke, which does not affect blood flow. This form of effleurage, shown at right below, follows nerve pathways and should be done from the head downward.

Effleurage is an excellent warm-up stroke: Start with a light variation and gradually work deeper. You will usually conclude your massage of each area with the nerve stroke, which is particularly soothing.

The broad surface of the back is ideal for practicing the five effleurage variations pictured here. Position yourself at the top of your partner's head and, starting at the base of his neck, stroke downward toward the waist. Use the muscles of your upper body, not just those of your arms and hands, to apply pressure evenly throughout the stroke. Keep your wrists flexible so your hands can adjust to your partner's changing body contours.

Release pressure at the bottom of his back and bring your hands back to the starting position, maintaining light contact with your fingertips. Stroke three times, moving approximately one to two inches per second and covering between 10 and 20 inches for the whole stroke. Do not apply any pressure on the spine.

BASIC EFFLEURAGE Position your hands close together, with your thumbs an inch or two apart *(opposite)*. Stroke downward, keeping your hands in firm contact with your partner's body.

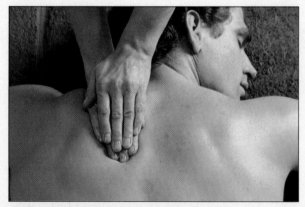
HAND ON HAND Place one hand on the other and glide your hands down the back near the spine.

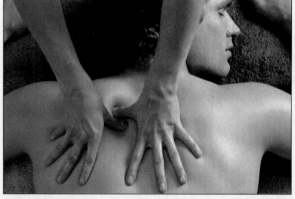
ADJACENT THUMB For deeper work, place one thumb next to the other and, using your fingers for support, glide down the back.

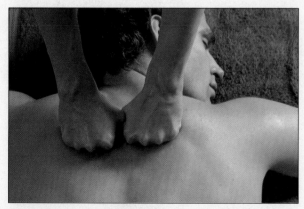
KNUCKLING For deep work on large muscles, make a fist and stroke with the midfinger joints.

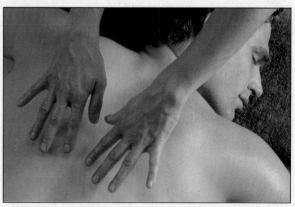
NERVE STROKE Brush the skin with your fingertips, or simply move your hands just above the skin without touching it.

Petrissage

A more complex technique than effleurage, petrissage progresses along a particular muscle group — usually on the limbs or a fleshy area where tissue is easily grasped. Like effleurage, petrissage can be performed either deeply or superficially. Deep petrissage is particularly effective at counteracting muscle atrophy, the tendency of muscles to degenerate from disuse. It does this by milking and draining the muscles through manual contraction and relaxation.

Petrissage is commonly called kneading, which aptly describes the way you should approach this movement — alternately tightening and loosening the hands (or fingers or thumbs) as they pick up and release muscle. Variations include rolling and wringing.

Note the changing musculature as you travel from the tendons and ligaments toward the belly, or center, of the muscle, which can usually withstand more pressure.

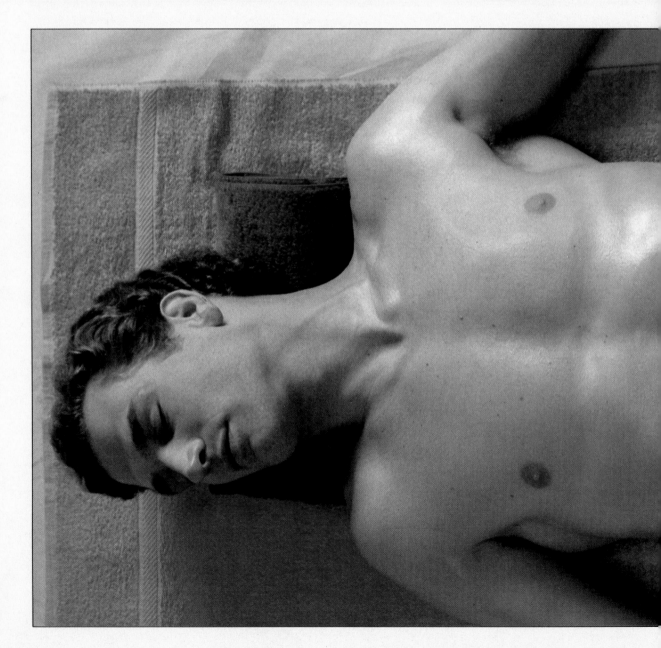

HAND ON HAND Use this stroke on broad or taut body surfaces. Place the fingers of your top hand over the bottom hand. Proceed in a clockwise direction, exerting even pressure.

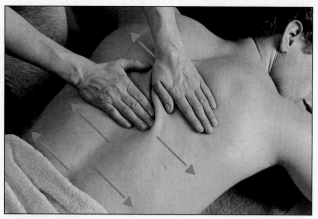

ROLLING Alternately slide your hands firmly back and forth across your partner's back. Start at shoulder level and move slightly lower with each stroke until you reach the waist.

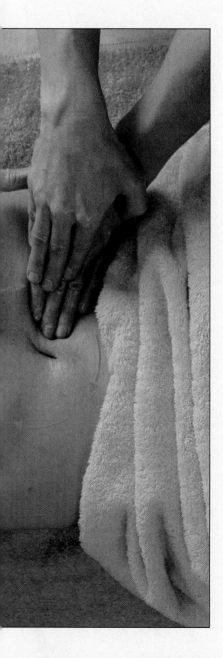

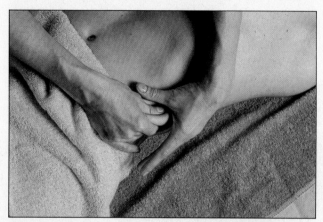

PICK UP Starting at your partner's waist, squeeze and release the skin first with your right hand, then with your left. Continue to alternate grasping and releasing as you progress up his side.

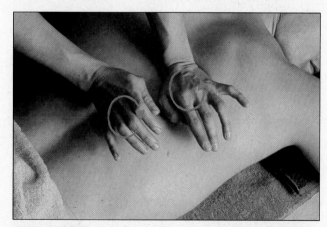

HEEL OF PALM Place the heels of your palms next to your partner's spine. Alternately rotating your palms in opposite directions, push the muscle gently away from his spine as you work down his back.

Friction

Movement into a joint is the key to friction. As in petrissage, you move muscle or soft tissue away from bone. But friction is a more specific stroke that is applied to a smaller area.

Because they have a relatively poor blood supply, tendons and ligaments are prime targets for injury and the formation of adhesions (matted clusters of muscular or connective-tissue fibers), particularly during exercise and sports activities. Friction, which increases circulation, works especially well to restore range of motion to joints by breaking down adhesions and softening scar tissue. For this reason, it is a mainstay of sports massage, where it is referred to as local cross-fiber stroking.

Use your fingertips and thumbs to perform friction; however, before you apply friction to sore areas, as athletic trainers often do, make sure your partner's physician approves. Then ask your partner to tell you how the friction feels; lighten pressure if he experiences undue discomfort. Friction should not be used on any recently injured tissue.

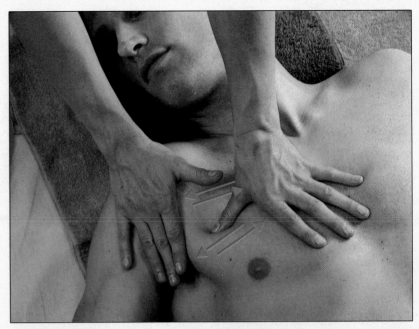

TRANSVERSE Place your thumbs parallel to each other where the shoulder and chest meet. Rapidly move them back and forth in opposite directions.

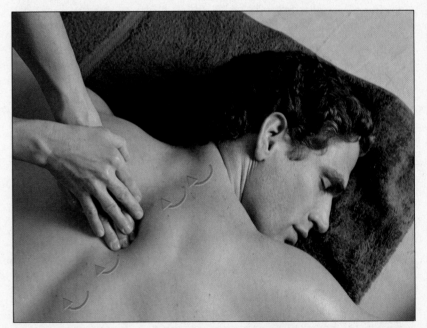

CIRCULAR FINGERTIP Place the fingertips of one hand next to your partner's spine. Put your other hand on top of the first and rotate your fingertips.

ONE THUMB Locate the ropelike tendons that join the shoulder to the back. Bracing your hand with your fingers, place your thumb on the tendons and rotate it in small circles.

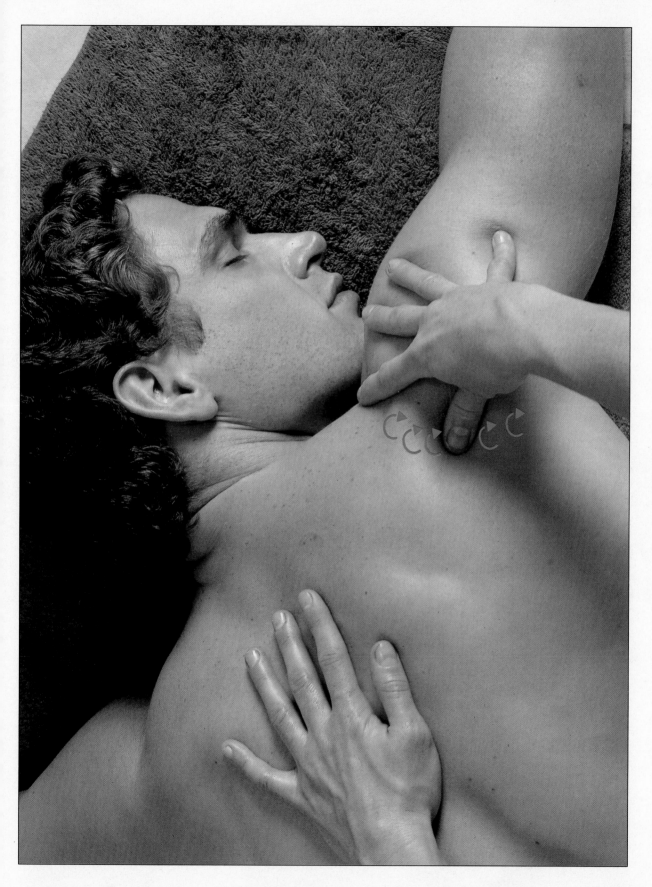

Percussion

Percussion strokes, also called tapotement (French for "tapping"), are alternate hand movements performed on broad areas of the body, particularly the back. There is some debate as to the deeper muscular benefits of percussion, but it is clearly beneficial in increasing surface blood circulation.

When performing percussion, keep your wrists relaxed and elbows flexed. Strike the skin with alternating hands, moving rapidly over the surface you are working on. You should strike firmly, but never so hard that you cause pain. And because even light percussion may cause discomfort to internal organs, you should not apply it on the lower abdomen, the lower back near the kidneys or the spine.

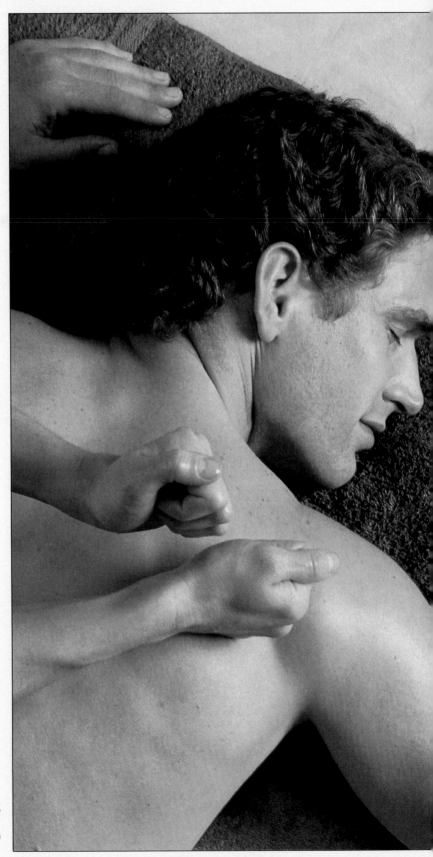

BEATING Form a loose fist and strike gently with the outside surface. Beating works best on the fleshier areas of the body, such as the shoulders, waist and thighs.

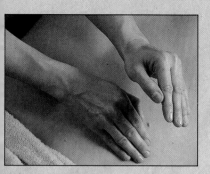

CUPPING Strike with your fingertips and the heels of your palms.

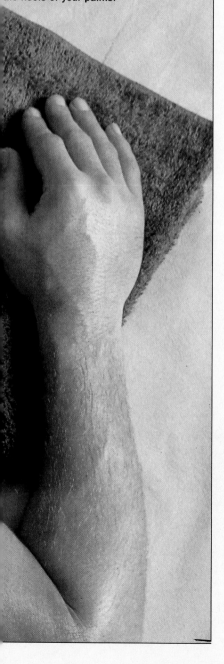

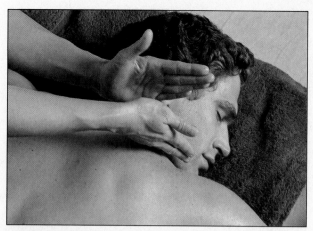

HACKING With the outer edge of your hands, perform light, rapid karate chops on fleshy areas like the upper shoulders.

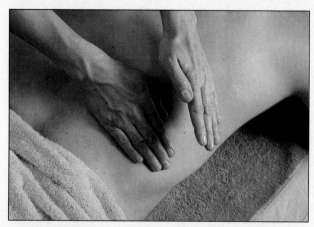

CLAPPING Flatten your hand and use the entire palm to clap rapidly over fleshy areas such as the waist.

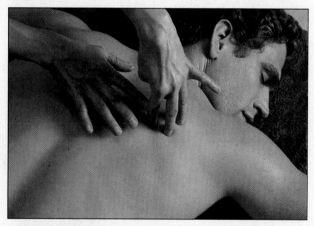

TAPPING Keeping your fingers straight, strike with the tips, alternating your hands quickly. Use this stroke on bony areas such as the shoulder blades.

Vibration and Jostling

These two techniques produce effects similar to percussion: They either stimulate or relax body tissue. Both strokes are particularly effective on the limbs and fleshy areas. Vibration does not proceed in any specific direction. Jostling, however, works up and down a particular muscle.

Vibration is tiring to perform, since it requires a rapid contraction and relaxation of your own muscles. This is why some professional massage therapists use mechanical vibrators. You can either follow their lead or keep vibrations to a minimum when you give a massage.

Jostling, which is not as strenuous to execute, plays an important role in sports massage, especially in treating sore muscles. While you are using other massage techniques, you may find your partner's muscles tensing up. This is called splinting, and it is a protective muscle reflex in response to pain or anticipation of pain. If this occurs, you can interrupt your sequence and relax the muscle area by jostling it for five to 10 seconds; then return to your routine. You can insert jostling into a massage as often as you want.

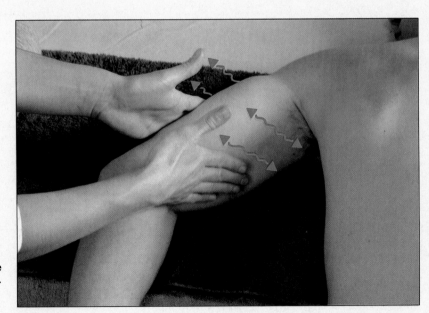

JOSTLING Place your hands on either side of your partner's biceps near the shoulder. Shake back and forth in a wavelike motion, progressing down the muscle.

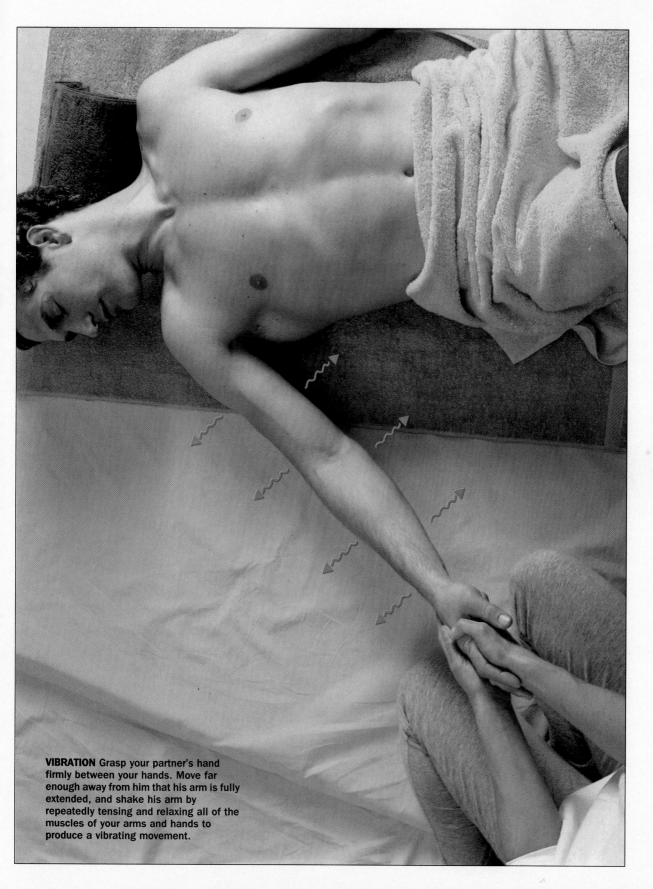

VIBRATION Grasp your partner's hand firmly between your hands. Move far enough away from him that his arm is fully extended, and shake his arm by repeatedly tensing and relaxing all of the muscles of your arms and hands to produce a vibrating movement.

Broad Cross-Fiber Stroking

Used primarily in sports massage, broad cross-fiber stroking stretches a muscle laterally, which breaks up existing adhesions deep in the muscle and prevents new adhesions from forming. It works more deeply into a muscle than petrissage, and it is extremely effective in treating fatigued or strained muscles.

Broad cross-fiber is a slow stroke that works only one or two muscle groups at a time. Align the outer surface of your thumb and palm with the length of the muscle, then roll your thumb across the grain of the muscle at a 90-degree angle.

Broad cross-fiber is usually performed in two directions, stroking first with one hand, then with the other. Pressure should be strong and consistent, coming from your entire arm, rather than from your wrist and hand. Deeper strokes are most effective, but some people will find them painful, so lighten the pressure if necessary.

When you perform the stroke, be aware of any point where the muscle does not roll easily. Repeat the stroke at such spots several times to help separate the muscle fibers.

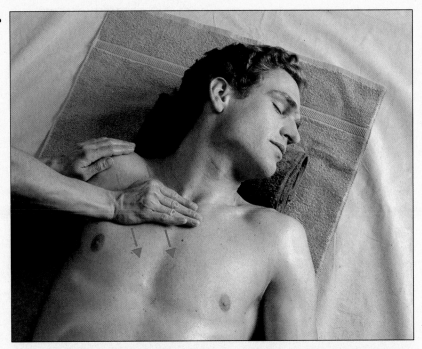

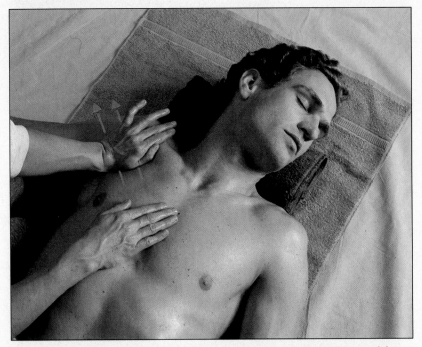

Place your left hand on your partner's right shoulder as a brace *(top)*. With your right thumb and palm, stroke diagonally down the chest. Then change hands. Use your right hand as a brace and stroke back to the shoulder with your left hand *(above)*.

Deep Stroking

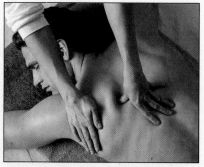

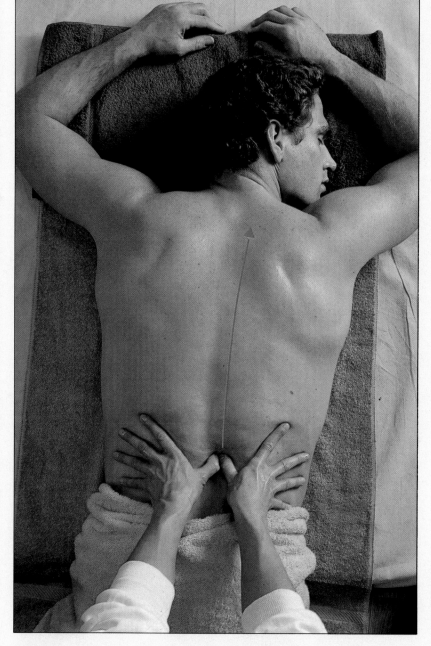

DOUBLE THUMB For added pressure, place one thumb on the other and glide.

ONE THUMB Use one thumb to glide deeply along smaller muscles.

The best massage movement for increasing blood flow to a particular area, deep stroking is actually a combination of effleurage and friction. Deep stroking glides along a muscle in the same direction as effleurage — toward the heart. But because it is performed deeply, it also serves some of the same functions as friction by greatly increasing circulation.

Work as deeply into the muscle tissue as possible without causing pain. Avoid the connective tissue — tendons and ligaments — where the muscle narrows, since heavy longitudinal strokes on those areas can cause tendinitis, a painful inflammation of the tendons.

JOINED THUMB Place your thumbs side by side along the erector muscles next to your partner's spine. Use your other fingers as a brace. Starting just below his waist, slide your thumbs up his back, pressing deeply into the muscle.

Compressions

The forceful strokes used in compression cause capillaries to dilate, creating a durable hyperemia, a large increase in blood supply that can cause a redness in the skin for up to 30 minutes. This circulation boost can benefit athletic performance, so compressions are frequently used in pre-exercise massage.

To perform the technique, use a rhythmic pumping motion, covering a muscle area with 30 to 40 compressions. Begin at the top of the area you are working and proceed around the entire musculature, avoiding bony areas such as the spine, knees and elbows. Keep your elbows slightly bent.

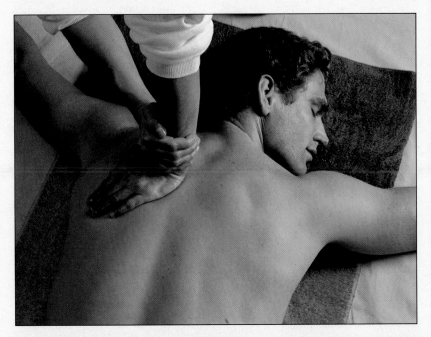

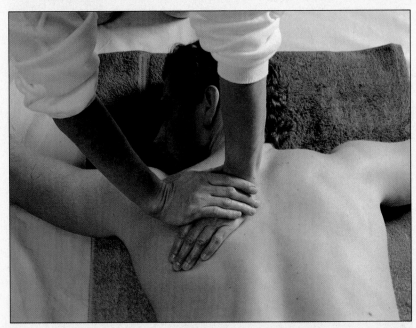

For smaller muscle areas, use one-hand pumping *(top)*: Place one palm flat on your partner's back, holding your wrist with your other hand for good leverage. Pump your hand up and down rapidly, gradually covering the back. For broad body surfaces, use hand-on-hand compressions *(above)*: Keep your hands pressed together while pumping.

Finger Pressure

In both shiatsu and trigger-point therapy, the basic technique is finger pressure. In shiatsu, you press *tsubos*, which correspond to acupuncture points. According to Eastern theory, these points line up along meridians, or energy channels, that run through the body, and pressing the points is believed to unblock and correct the body's flow of energy. *(For more on shiatsu theory, see pages 72-75.)*

Trigger points are painful spots in a muscle that stem from a variety of causes, including birth trauma, sports injuries and daily stress. When trigger points flare up, they cause muscle spasms, which reduce the blood supply to a specific area. The continued muscle contraction produced by the spasm leads to a build-up of lactic acid that, combined with the reduced blood flow, causes the area to become hypersensitive.

As you give a massage, you will be able to detect trigger points: The build-up of crystallized metabolic by-products, particularly lactic acid, makes them feel like small marbles. Because of the hypersensitivity associated with trigger points, your partner may complain of pain or involuntarily tense his muscles when you touch these spots.

When you locate a trigger point, apply pressure with your thumb for up to 15 seconds. This will break up the crystallized substances, releasing them into the bloodstream.

Sometimes the trigger point is so sensitive that you will have to use repeated treatments of increasing intensity to eliminate it. After the pain subsides, your partner will feel a release of tension as blood flow returns to normal in the affected area.

To apply pressure for either trigger points or shiatsu, use the ball of your thumb. Extend your thumb in a smooth line from your hand, using your fingers as a base. Apply pressure steadily, without rubbing.

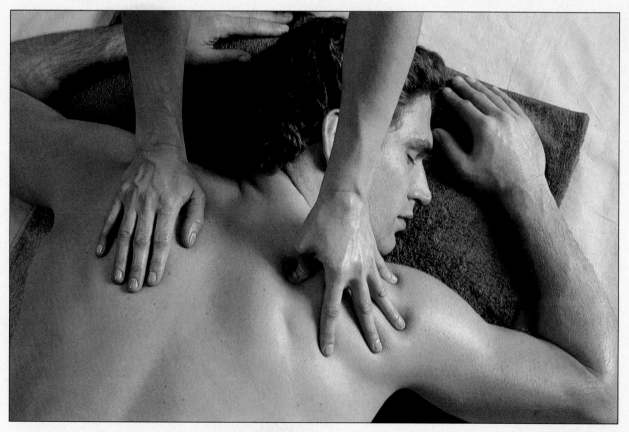

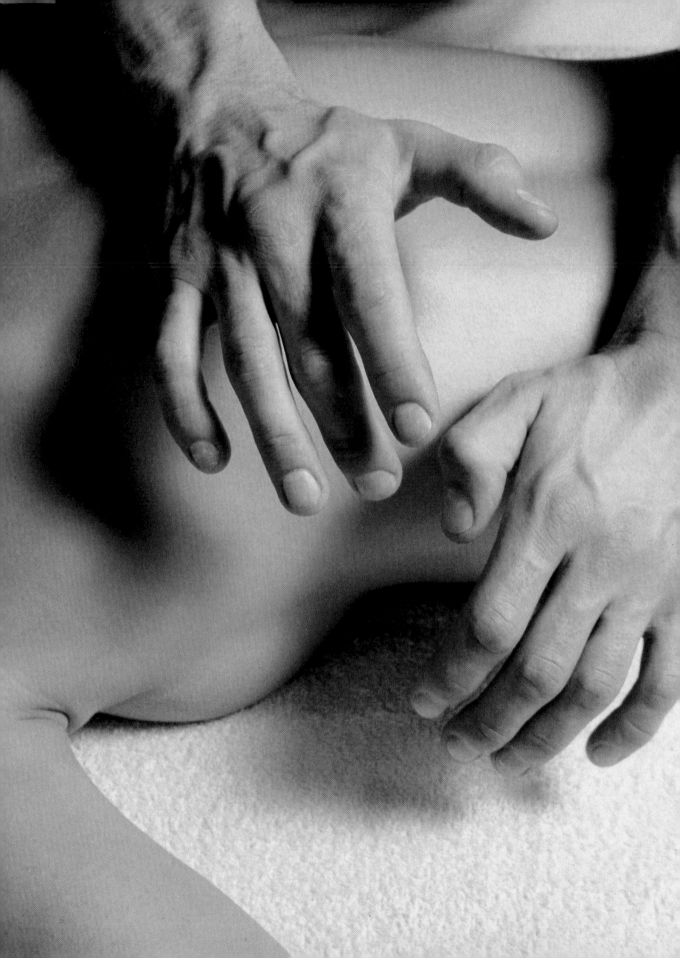

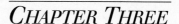

CHAPTER THREE

Full-Body Massage

*The best of Eastern and Western
techniques, step by step*

Once you have learned the basic techniques covered in the previous chapter, you can combine them systematically to massage nearly all the muscles in the body. Creating the right environment for a massage is the first step toward making the experience pleasant. Since the primary goal is relaxation, you should eliminate any distractions that might disturb your partner or interfere with your concentration as you give the massage.

The room you work in should be warm, since areas of your partner's skin will be exposed during the massage. Cool or chilly air may not only feel unpleasant, but can also cause the muscles to contract, thereby reducing the effectiveness of the massage. An ideal temperature is between 72 and 74 degrees Fahrenheit. Make sure that your hands are warm, too, before you touch your partner; if necessary, rub them together vigorously to heat them. Proper draping *(see box page 49)* will also help keep your partner warm.

Lighting should be soft; avoid bright overhead or fluorescent lights.

47

If you and your partner enjoy background music, choose quiet selections that will contribute to the soothing, relaxing mood of the massage. Many massage therapists actually favor "white noise" machines that produce constant, nondistracting background sounds.

The techniques in this chapter are shown on a table, but you can apply them just as effectively on the floor — indeed, shiatsu is traditionally done on the floor. When massaging on the floor, though, be careful to bend your back as little as possible to avoid straining it. Kneeling on pillows will help alleviate knee discomfort. Whether you are using a massage table or the floor, be sure to cover the surface with a clean sheet.

The following pages present several options for a full-body massage. You can give a massage that relies for the most part on Swedish techniques *(pages 50-71)*. Or you can concentrate on shiatsu or reflexology, two Eastern-based techniques *(pages 72-79)*. When you have developed proficiency with various strokes, you might choose to blend these techniques, as many professional massage therapists do. For example, you can incorporate the shiatsu pressure points called *tsubos* into Swedish massage. This chapter also offers a comprehensive self-massage routine that includes a special section on cosmetic massage *(pages 80-93)*.

Before starting, have your partner remove glasses or contact lenses and all jewelry. He or she should initially lie prone, with the top of his or her head about even with the end of the table or the padding on the floor. Begin a full-body massage on your partner's back. Because you want to keep any effort or movement by your partner to a minimum, you should complete all your work on the back of the body before asking your partner to turn over. On both the back and the front of the body, massage should proceed from the top of the body down the trunk, finishing with the limbs.

Work one area of the body completely, then move on to an adjacent area. For example, follow massage on the back with work on the buttocks and then the legs. When moving from one part of your partner's body to another, use connecting strokes — a long effleurage or nerve stroke — to make the transition. After your final strokes on the chest, for example, do a light effleurage from the chest to the abdomen to signal to your partner that you will be working on that area next.

The order of strokes on any particular part of the body is somewhat arbitrary. Except where noted, you should always begin with a long effleurage and end with some variation of percussion, followed by a final broad effleurage and then a nerve stroke. Massage strokes are given in multiples of three, so that you perform each stroke three, six or occasionally nine times. As you become more proficient at massage, you might want to vary the order of the strokes shown here, or you may prefer to concentrate longer on an area that your partner especially enjoys having massaged.

The amount of pressure you should use is determined partly by the

How to Drape Your Partner

◆ Draping is an important aspect of full-body massage that meets both emotional and physical needs of your partner. Proper draping — leaving exposed only the part of the body you are working on — can alleviate your partner's sensitivity about undressing, as well as avoid possible physical discomfort. Having his or her body exposed can make your partner feel vulnerable and possibly create anxiety, thereby reducing the relaxing benefits of the massage. Also, while the area of the body you are working on will be warmed by the strokes, other parts, particularly the hands and feet, can easily become chilled. In addition, oil makes the body more temperature-sensitive.

◆ The warmth of the room where you are massaging determines how heavily you will drape your partner. You should have both sheets and blankets on hand. To start, place a large sheet over the massage table or surface, allowing it to hang over the sides. Have your partner lie face down and snugly wrap both sides of the sheet over him or her. Open the sheet from the top, just enough to expose your partner's back. When you finish massaging the back and buttocks, close the sheet; then open it from the bottom to expose one leg. If your partner is chilly, add a blanket. Because your partner is partially clothed for shiatsu and reflexology, draping is unnecessary, although a blanket may be necessary if he or she becomes cold.

◆ After you have completed massaging the back of the body, your partner will turn over. At this time, professional massage therapists hold up the side of the sheet nearest them, covering their partner's body as soon as he or she turns over. Depending on your relationship with your massage partner, such efforts to preserve your partner's modesty may not be necessary.

stroke and partly by your partner. Generally, you should apply as much pressure as your partner can withstand, as he or she will derive greater benefits from the massage if you work deeply into the muscles. But let up if your partner gives any indication of pain, either verbally or by tensing the muscles you are massaging. Sometimes you can work through the pain with breathing: Have your partner breathe deeply and synchronize your breathing with his. Exert pressure as you both exhale. Also, keep your nails trimmed, since long nails can cause pain.

Ticklishness is another problem you may encounter when giving a massage, particularly on the feet and abdomen. If this occurs, have your partner concentrate on breathing and use deeper pressure.

Any soreness your partner feels during or immediately after the massage is due to the release of metabolic by-products like uric acid and lactic acid into the bloodstream; the soreness should disappear within an hour or so. More likely, your partner will be in a deep state of relaxation; some people even fall asleep during a massage. If this happens, proceed as usual, and let him or her rest quietly for several minutes after you have completed the massage.

Upper Back

It is understandable that many people equate a massage with a back rub. The muscles that support the back are often subjected to tension or strain, typically from sitting or standing for long periods or from poor posture. Massaging these muscles can impart an overall sense of relaxation. And because most people have had a back rub, someone who is initially uncomfortable about receiving a full-body massage is more likely to relax when you start with the back.

The techniques you should use are divided into upper back routines, shown on these two pages, and lower back routines, illustrated on the following two pages. But you should handle the back as a unit, using connecting strokes to link the two areas.

Stand at your partner's side with one hand on her right shoulder blade and the other hand at her left hip. Perform a spinal stretch by pressing outward with your arms as you and your partner exhale. Repeat twice, then perform the same sequence with your hands reversed.

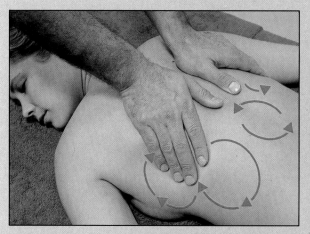
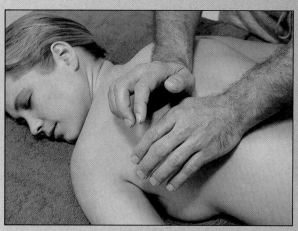

Stand at your partner's head. Effleurage down her back six times, then effleurage outward to her side in overlapping, fanning circles that progress down her entire back. Perform the whole sequence three times.

Place the heels of your palms on the far side of your partner's spine and petrissage in opposing circles down her back. Perform three times, then perform three times on the other side of her back, now pulling toward you.

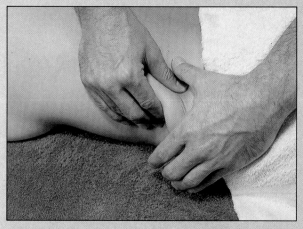
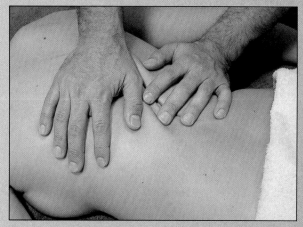

Reach across your partner's body and use alternate hands to rhythmically pick up from the waist to under her arms. Perform three times, switch sides, then perform three times on the other side of her back.

Place your hands flat on your partner's back and do a rolling petrissage. Work from the top of the back down to the waist, then back up, covering the entire width with each cross stroke. Perform three times.

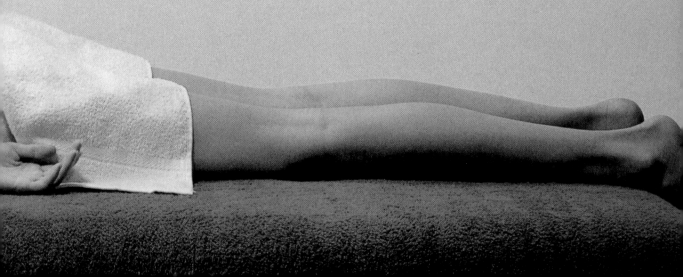

Lower Back and Buttocks

The largest muscle of the back, the latissimus dorsi, extends from the lower back all the way to the armpit. Because of its breadth, the latissimus is often inadequately and unevenly stretched, causing it to shorten and tighten. This is a common cause of lower back pain.

Whether or not your partner suffers from lower back pain or tension, massage will help keep the muscles in the area relaxed. This can decrease the likelihood of a back flare-up and can ease any existing pain.

Massage to the buttocks focuses attention on an often-overlooked muscle group that you use each time you take a step. Strain to the buttocks can lead to pain in the lower back and legs, so keeping these large and powerful muscles relaxed indirectly benefits adjacent muscles as well.

When massaging this area, straddle your partner so that you are kneeling just below the buttocks. This will give you the leverage you need to work deeply on these muscles. Finish the back massage with an effleurage over the entire back, followed by a nerve stroke.

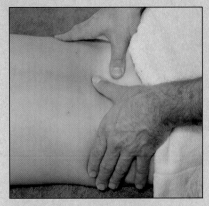

Circular-thumb petrissage across the large triangular bone at the base of the spine. (Do not massage elsewhere on the spine.)

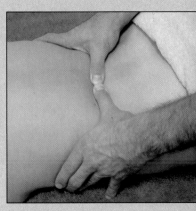

Use joined-thumb effleurage on one side of the spine from the waist to the neck. Perform three times; switch sides.

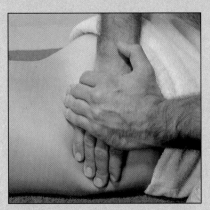

Use hand-on-hand effleurage to stroke outward from the center of the buttocks. Perform six times, then switch sides.

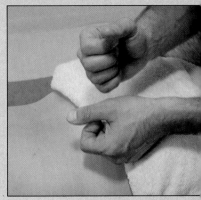

Use loose fists to drum lightly on the gluteals for 10 seconds. Work up the back, avoiding the kidney area and the spine.

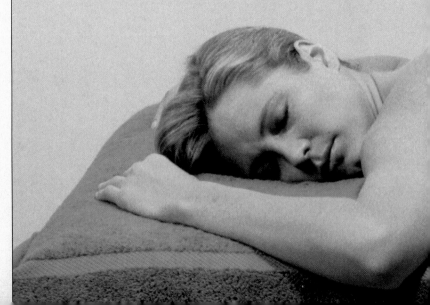

Start at the buttocks and, with your fingertips, effleurage the entire back up to the neck. This will connect the work on the lower and upper back. Glide back down. Perform this sequence three times.

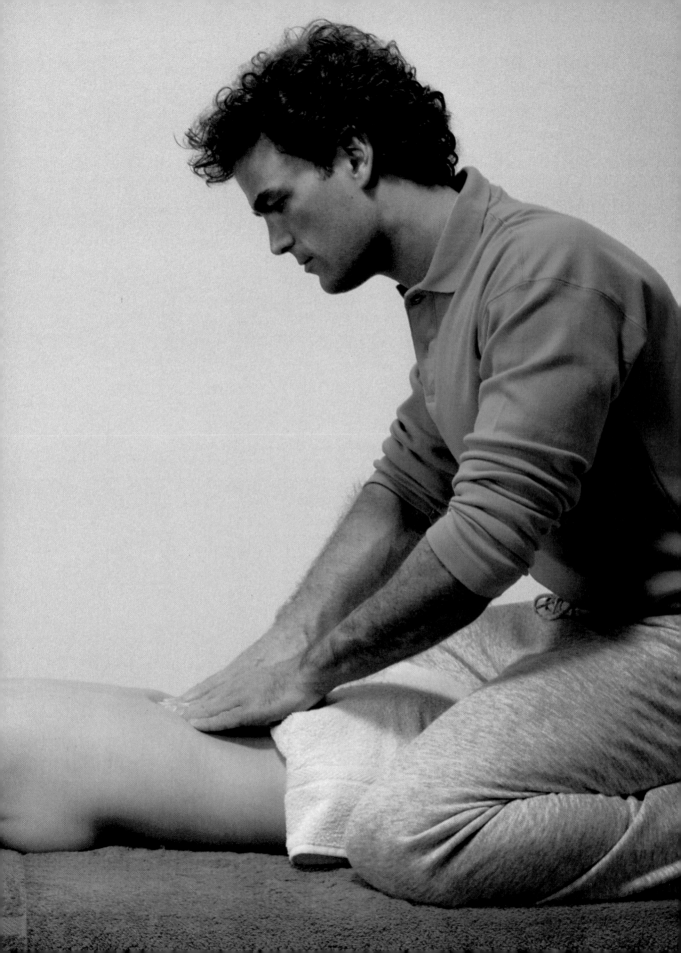

Posterior Leg

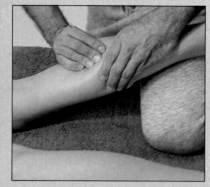

Perform circular-thumb petrissage from the ankle to the hip. Do three times.

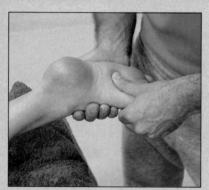

Pick up from the calf to the thigh, working along the inner thigh. Perform three times.

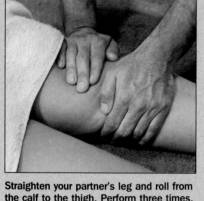

Straighten your partner's leg and roll from the calf to the thigh. Perform three times.

Apply small circular petrissage on the bottom of the entire foot.

Massaging the back of your partner's legs will complete your work on the back of her body. Start by applying oil with a long, basic effleurage. Work up from the ankle to the buttocks and glide back down to the foot. You may wish to prop your partner's ankle on your bent leg to give you more leverage.

Complete the massage of each leg with a broad effleurage and a nerve stroke. To maintain the continuity of the strokes, do the entire routine on one leg before moving on to the other. When massaging the legs, avoid deep pressure on the back of the knees or on varicose veins.

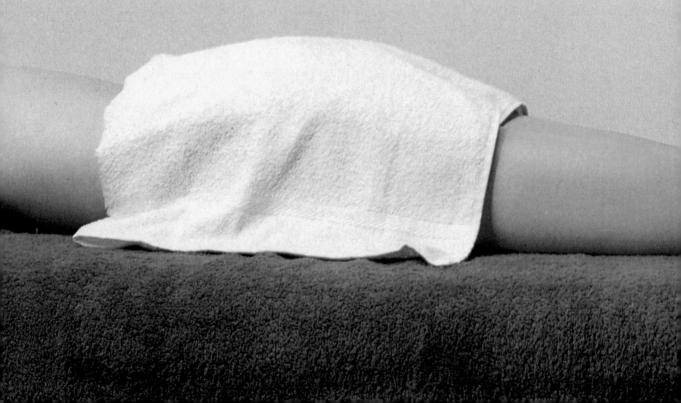

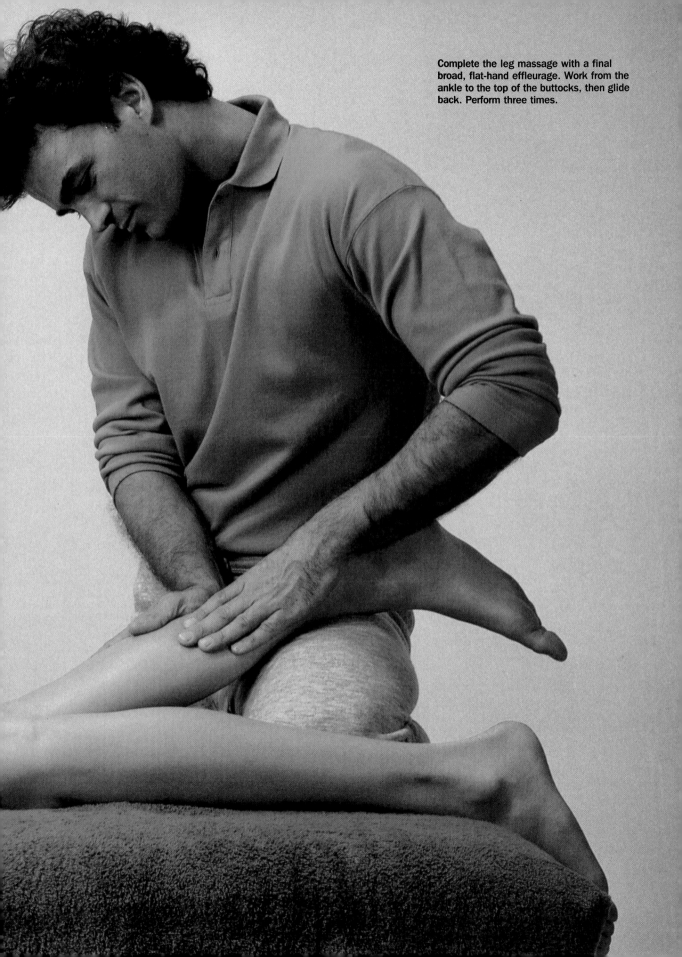

Complete the leg massage with a final broad, flat-hand effleurage. Work from the ankle to the top of the buttocks, then glide back. Perform three times.

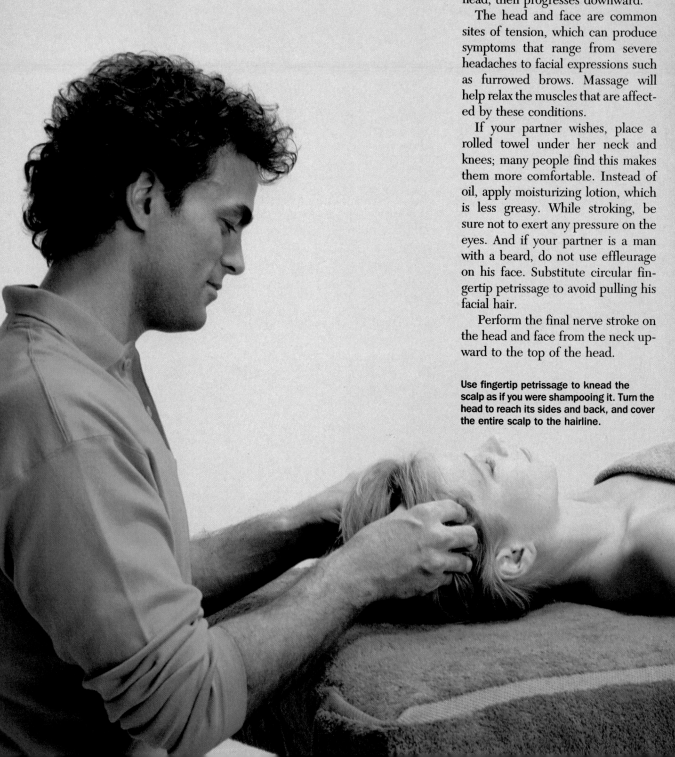

Head and Face

After you have finished massaging the back of your partner's legs, ask her to turn over. A massage of the front of the body begins with the face and head, then progresses downward.

The head and face are common sites of tension, which can produce symptoms that range from severe headaches to facial expressions such as furrowed brows. Massage will help relax the muscles that are affected by these conditions.

If your partner wishes, place a rolled towel under her neck and knees; many people find this makes them more comfortable. Instead of oil, apply moisturizing lotion, which is less greasy. While stroking, be sure not to exert any pressure on the eyes. And if your partner is a man with a beard, do not use effleurage on his face. Substitute circular fingertip petrissage to avoid pulling his facial hair.

Perform the final nerve stroke on the head and face from the neck upward to the top of the head.

Use fingertip petrissage to knead the scalp as if you were shampooing it. Turn the head to reach its sides and back, and cover the entire scalp to the hairline.

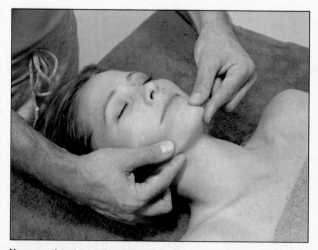

Use your thumb and forefinger for a fingertip effleurage from the center of the chin to the ears; do three times. Perform a fingertip effleurage from the side of the nose across the cheekbones.

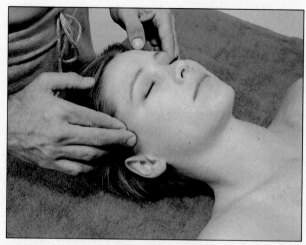

Place the first two fingers of each hand at your partner's temples. Rotate in a circular petrissage, pressing lightly on the temples for eight to 10 seconds.

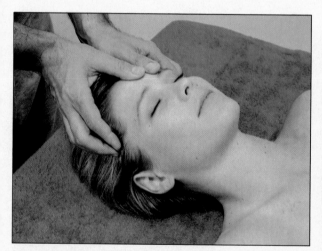

Grasp your partner's head lightly with both hands and place your thumbs on her forehead so they point to her nose. Move them up and down in a transverse friction. Cover her forehead three times.

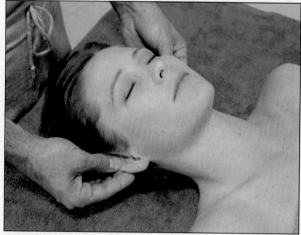

Hold your partner's outer ears between your thumb and forefinger. Rub each ear by moving your fingers back and forth; work down the ear and then back up.

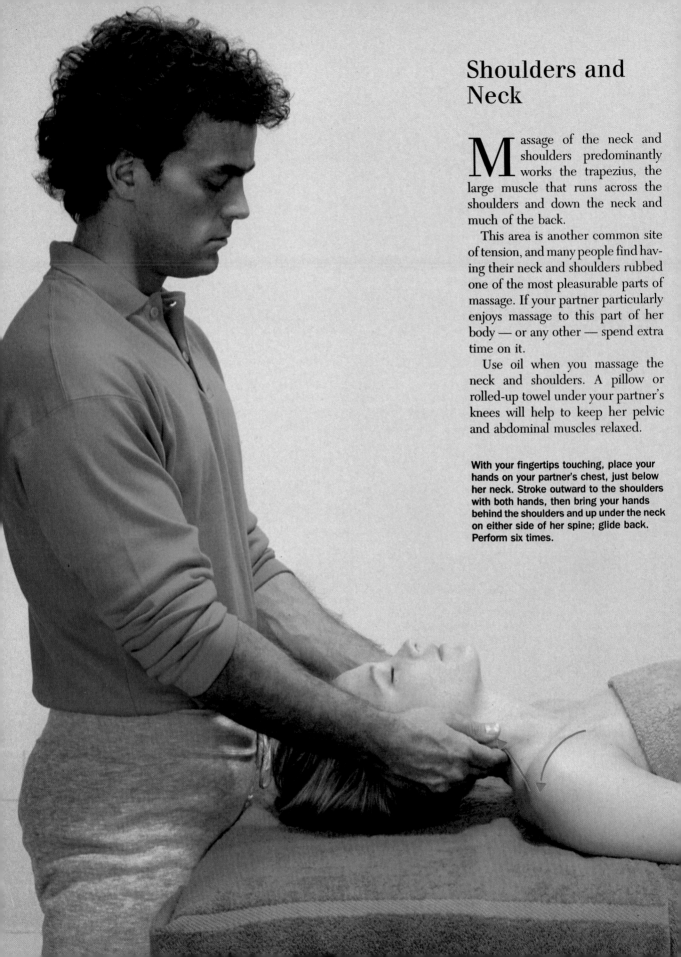

Shoulders and Neck

Massage of the neck and shoulders predominantly works the trapezius, the large muscle that runs across the shoulders and down the neck and much of the back.

This area is another common site of tension, and many people find having their neck and shoulders rubbed one of the most pleasurable parts of massage. If your partner particularly enjoys massage to this part of her body — or any other — spend extra time on it.

Use oil when you massage the neck and shoulders. A pillow or rolled-up towel under your partner's knees will help to keep her pelvic and abdominal muscles relaxed.

With your fingertips touching, place your hands on your partner's chest, just below her neck. Stroke outward to the shoulders with both hands, then bring your hands behind the shoulders and up under the neck on either side of her spine; glide back. Perform six times.

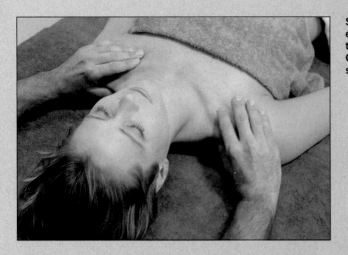

Start just above the base of the neck and effleurage down the neck and across the top of the shoulders with your thumbs. Glide back with your thumbs. Perform this sequence three times.

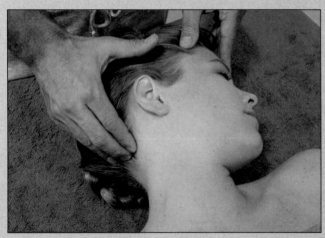

Turn your partner's head to one side. Start next to her spine at the base of her neck and use circular fingertip friction to work up her neck and along the edge of the scalp. Perform three times, then switch sides.

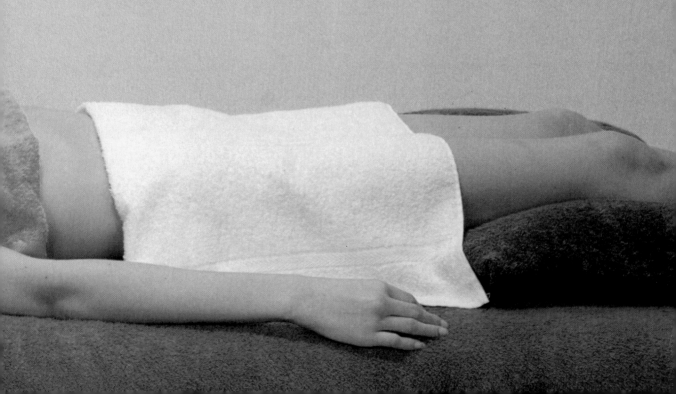

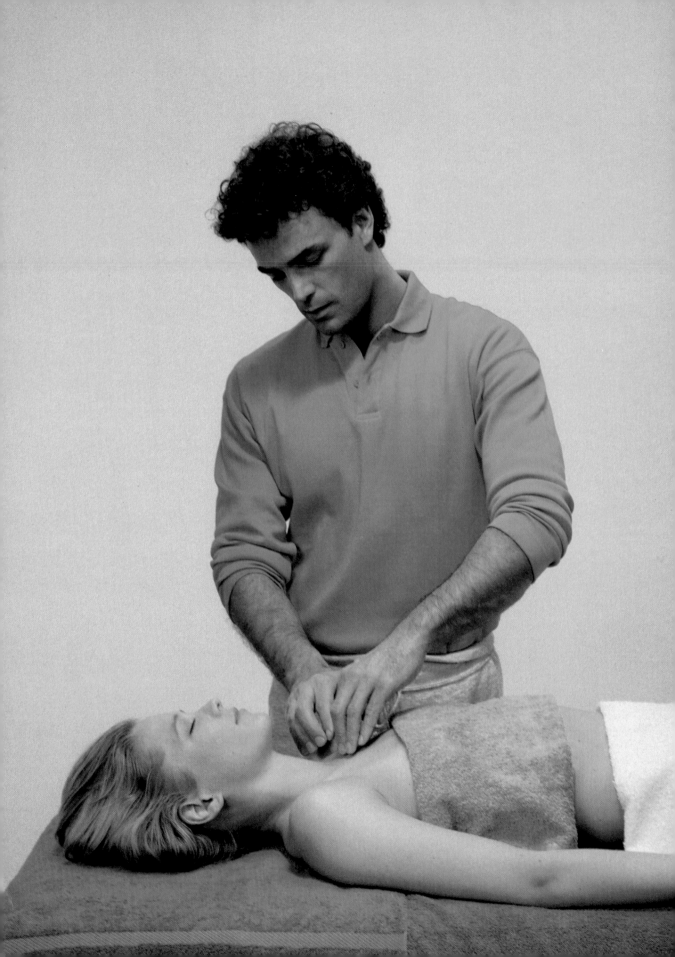

Chest

The pectoralis major, the large two-part muscle that spans the chest, affects both breathing and upper body alignment. Because this muscle expands and contracts with every breath, any tightness can restrict breathing. Tension in the chest muscles also affects the adjacent muscles of the back and neck, massaging the chest can relax the entire area.

Chest massage differs for men and women. If your partner is a woman, do not exert any direct pressure on her breasts; instead, work around and between the breasts, using more petrissage than effleurage. Finish any chest massage with a nerve stroke.

Stand at your partner's side or head. Tap lightly with alternate fingers over the surface of your partner's chest. This percussion can be done on the bony areas of the chest.

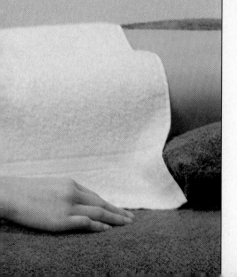

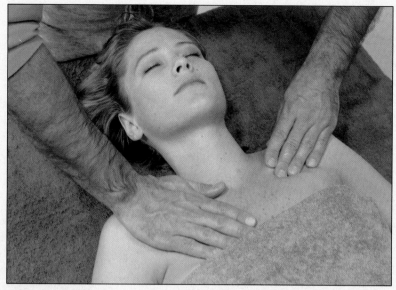

Move to your partner's head. Work alternately from her shoulder toward the center of her chest, using a flat-hand effleurage. Perform three times.

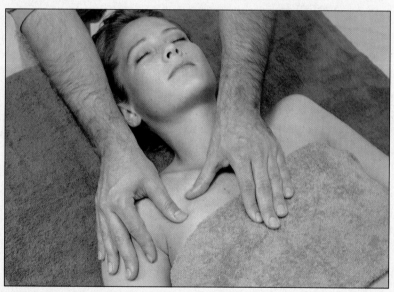

Start at your partner's shoulder and alternate thumbs to knead downward. Progress toward the middle of the chest, then switch sides.

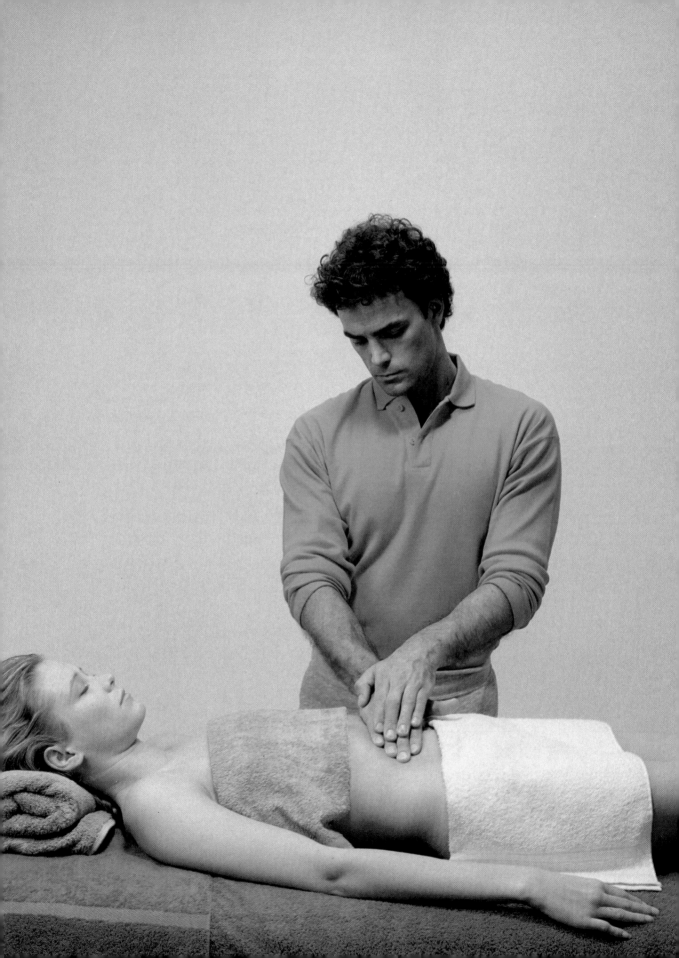

The Midsection/1

Many people initially feel uneasy during massage to their abdomen. A soothing way to begin work on this region is with the strokes shown here, which are derived from shiatsu and are targeted at the *hara* (Japanese for "abdomen"). In shiatsu, the hara refers to an area located a hand's breadth below the navel. It is considered the body's center of energy, and while strengthening the hara with shiatsu helps the whole body, the abdomen and the back receive the greatest benefit.

Begin with very gentle pressure and keep your movements smooth and gradual. Deep pressure should not be used on the abdomen to avoid possible damage to internal organs. Continue with the Swedish strokes shown on the following two pages. Always work clockwise around the abdomen to stimulate the digestion, which travels in that direction in the large intestine.

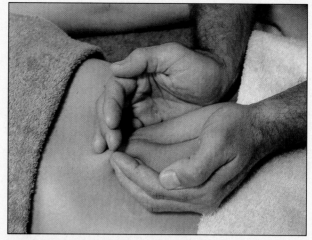

Cup your hands around your partner's navel. As she exhales, gently press down into the abdomen and squeeze your hands together slightly. Rotate your hands clockwise and repeat twice.

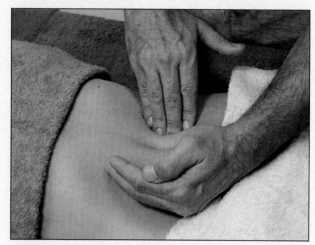

Keep your left hand cupped around your partner's navel. On exhalation, gently press the near side of the navel with the fingers of your right hand. Move clockwise, alternating hands to complete a full rotation.

Stand or kneel at your partner's side. With one hand on top of the other, cover her navel. Rock your hands back and forth from the fingertips to the heel of the palm in a continuous wavelike motion. Do nine times.

The Midsection/2

Place your hands, one on top of the other, on your partner's right side under her ribs. Gently vibrate the heel of your palm by tensing and shaking the muscles in your arms and hands. Repeat on her left side.

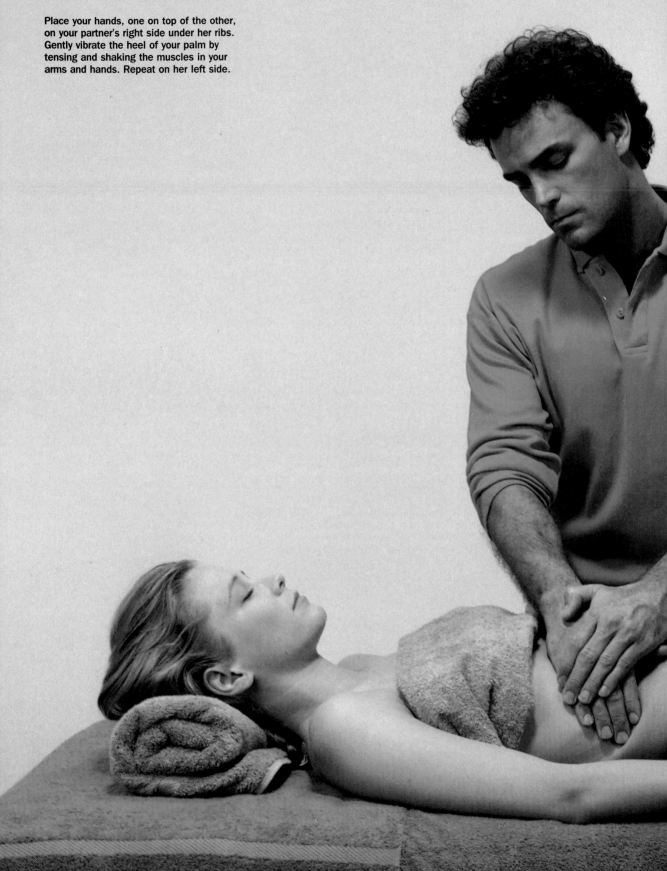

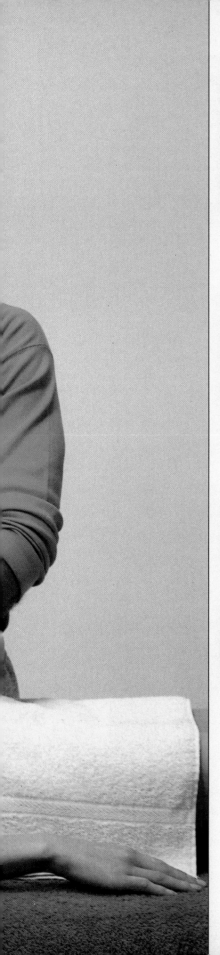

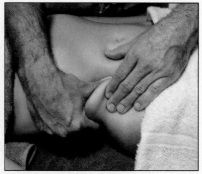

Reach across your partner and pick up at her side. Work up from the hips to the ribs, then back down. Perform three times.

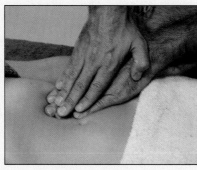

Use circular-fingertip petrissage to work clockwise from the lower right abdomen to the lower left.

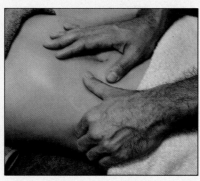

Use alternate-thumb petrissage to work clockwise around the abdomen. Circle the abdomen three times.

Arms

The arms contain numerous muscles and tendons in a relatively small space. Many of these muscles, like the biceps and the opposing triceps, are repeatedly exercised in everyday activities. Continual use places pressure on the adjoining tendons; this can lead to muscular aches and decreased range of motion in the arm. Massaging the arm will help restore range of motion to the joints.

Perform each of the strokes shown here three times. Be sure to use only light pressure over the elbow and shoulder — a network of tendons makes these joints especially sensitive. After you complete the entire routine on one arm, pull the arm away from the body and vibrate it. Do a final effleurage and nerve stroke, then repeat the sequence on the other arm.

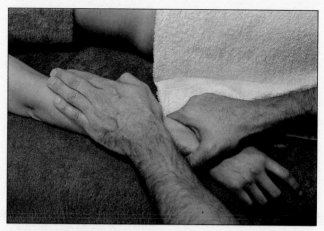

Hold your partner's arm palm down with one hand. Effleurage from the wrist to the shoulder with your other hand, then turn the arm palm up and effleurage along the inside.

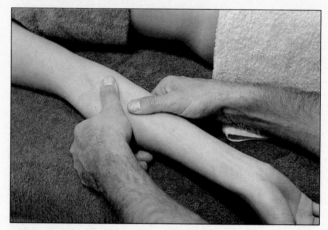

Keep your partner's arm palm up. Work up the arm from the wrist, using alternate-thumb petrissage. Use your fingers to support the arm from underneath.

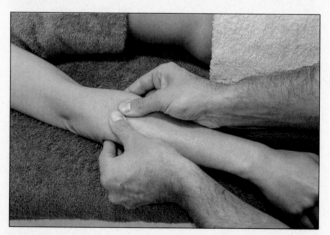

Use joined-thumb effleurage on the outside of the arm, working from the wrist to the shoulder. Position your fingers underneath the arm to serve as a brace.

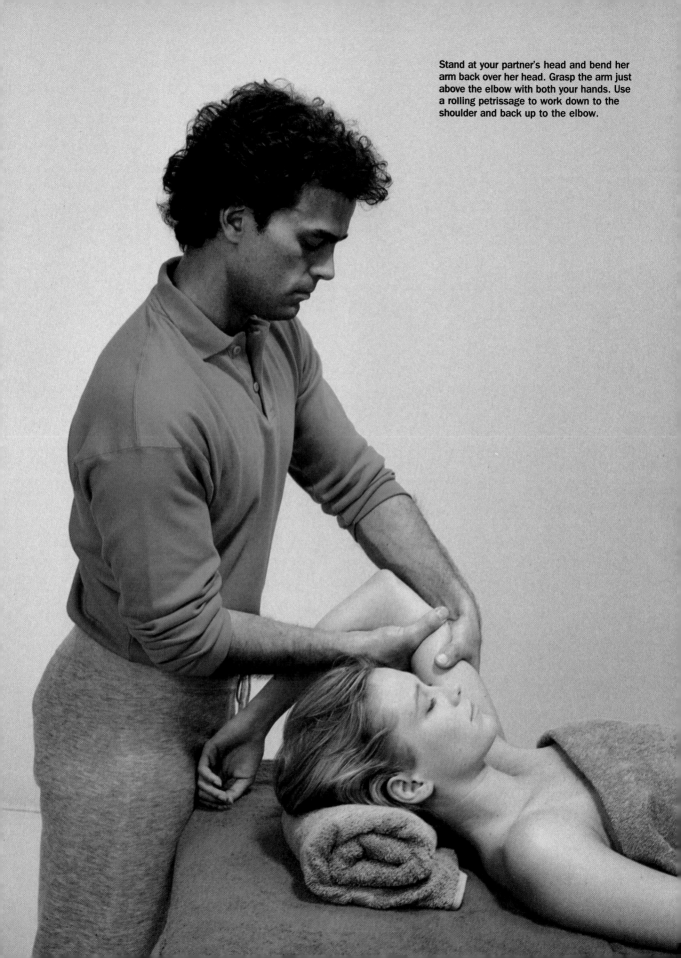

Stand at your partner's head and bend her arm back over her head. Grasp the arm just above the elbow with both your hands. Use a rolling petrissage to work down to the shoulder and back up to the elbow.

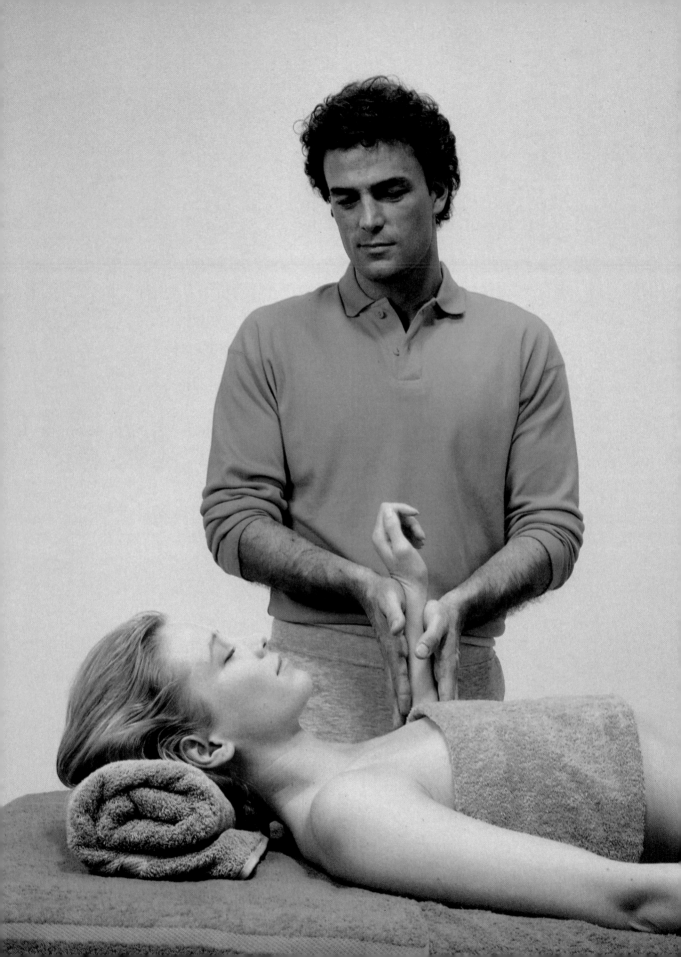

Hands

You use your hands virtually every waking minute of every day. Due to the demands placed on them and their complex structure, your hands are vulnerable to a range of problems as minor as cramps and as debilitating as arthritis. The hand contains a relatively large number of joints and tendons — more than 15 tendons connect it to the forearm. A massage can relax the hands, increase circulation and restore range of motion.

Its many small bones and muscles make some massage strokes unsuitable for the hand. Therefore, much of the routine shown here uses friction to work tendons and joints. Perform the entire routine on one hand, then repeat it on the other one.

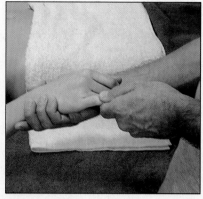

Rub each of your partner's fingers between your thumb and finger. Work from the knuckles to the tips.

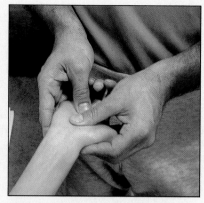

Hold your partner's hand palm up in your hands. Work across the palm with a circular-thumb petrissage.

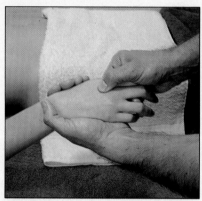

Turn her hand palm down again. Hold it with one hand and do one-thumb friction between her hand bones with your other.

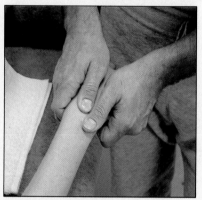

Move your thumbs back and forth in transverse friction on the outside of the wrist; repeat on the inside.

Bend your partner's arm up, keeping her elbow resting on the table or floor. Grasp her arm between both of yours so that your palms are at her wrist. Move your hands rapidly up and down in a broad friction; the motion should cause your partner's hand to flop back and forth with a slapping sound.

Anterior Leg

Complete the full-body massage by working the front of your partner's leg. You will be able to apply more pressure and broader strokes on the large muscles of the leg, especially the thigh, than you have on the rest of the front of the body.

Move to your partner's feet and start with a long effleurage on the outside of the leg, working from the ankle to the hip. Lighten pressure at the knee, as at all bony areas.

After executing the strokes shown here, use circular-fingertip friction around the ankle, then effleurage over the top of the ankle and work the toes much as you did the fingers on the preceding pages. *(For more on foot massage and reflexology, see pages 76-79.)* Finally, hold your partner's leg at the ankle and do a vibration, followed by another effleurage and return nerve stroke.

Conclude your full-body massage with a nerve stroke done just over — but not quite touching — the entire front of the body, from the top of the head to slightly beyond the feet.

Stand at your partner's feet and place your hands on either side of her leg *(below).* **Work up the leg, using your palms for broad, circular petrissage.**

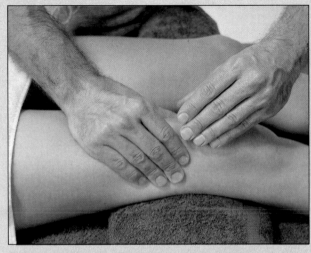

Stand at your partner's thigh and do a pick-up petrissage, working from the calf to the top of the thigh. Avoid the knee and hip joints. Repeat twice. Then do a rolling petrissage up and down the thigh.

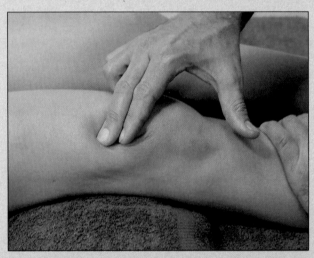

Bend your partner's knee slightly and use your first two fingers for circular friction across the tendons just above the kneecap. Repeat on the ligaments just below the knee.

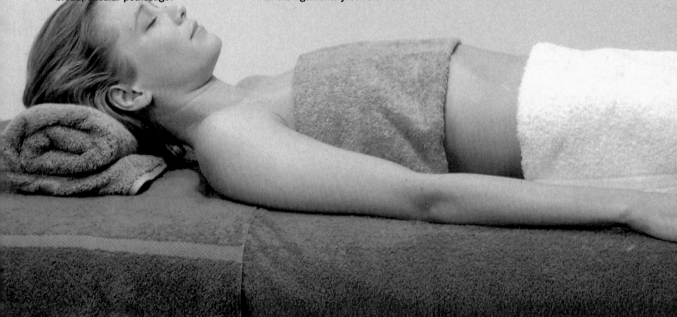

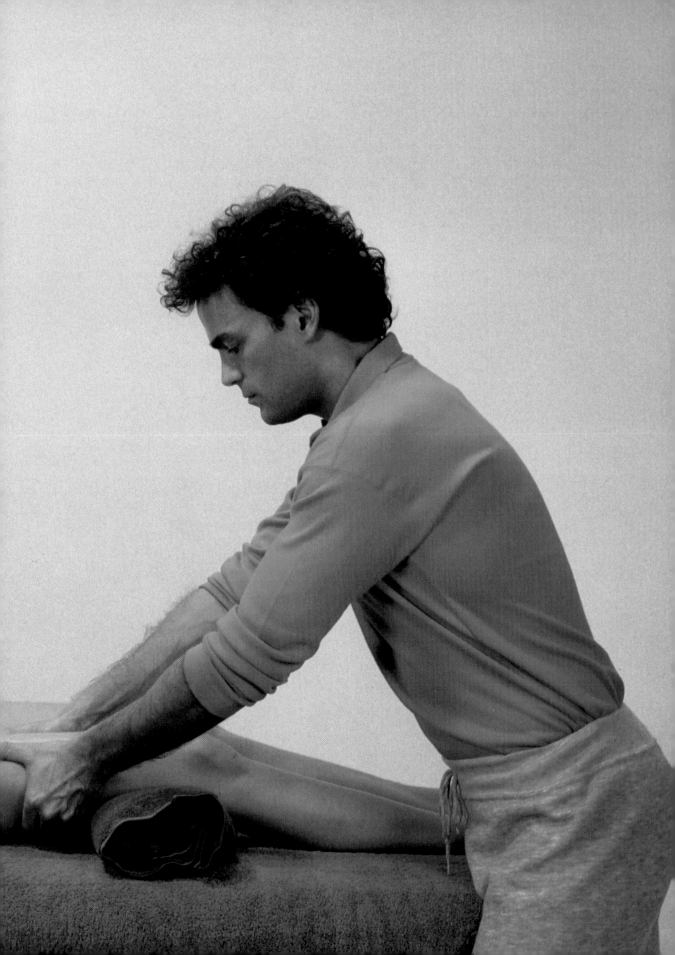

Shiatsu/1

The ancient Japanese pressure-point therapy called shiatsu is based on the belief that a vital energy, or *ki*, circulates through our bodies along pathways called meridians. In the physiology of shiatsu — which, although widely practiced, has not been verified experimentally — there are 14 major meridians, each corresponding to a specific organ or physical or mental function.

Tsubos are points along the meridians where you can most easily make contact with *ki*. Many of the *tsubos* correspond to trigger points used in Western massage systems.

Ideally, *ki* flows smoothly through the meridians to keep the body in peak condition. But mental or physical tension, injury or illness can disrupt this energy flow. In shiatsu, this flow is restored — and any related conditions, such as headaches, are corrected — by pressing the appropriate *tsubo*.

Basic shiatsu is simple to perform. It requires only a simple pressing technique, shown on page 45, which is applied to the *tsubos*, usually with your fingers or thumbs. You should perform shiatsu on a padded or carpeted floor. Have your partner wear loose, comfortable clothing and do not use oil.

You usually apply shiatsu from a kneeling position. Lean in with your body to exert pressure, using your arms for support. Bend your elbows slightly and keep both hands in contact with your partner's body. Press each *tsubo* for five to 10 seconds. If your partner feels pain, ease the pressure.

Apply pressure to the muscles along both sides of the spine, then press the *tsubos* shown here. The *tsubos* for the front of the body are shown on the following two pages.

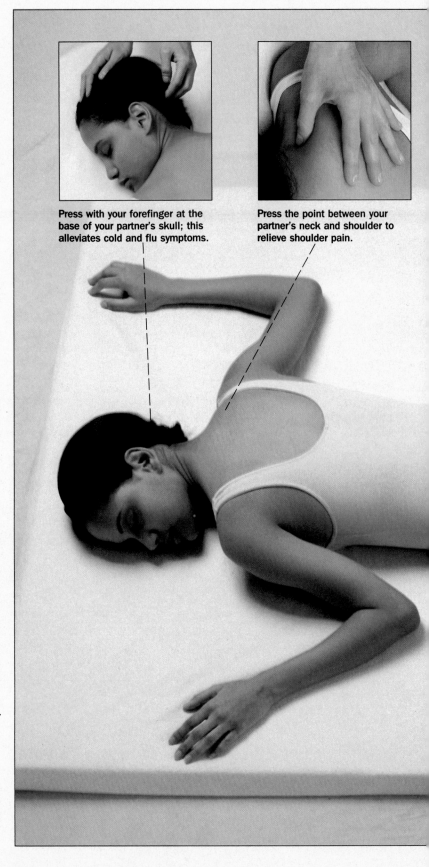

Press with your forefinger at the base of your partner's skull; this alleviates cold and flu symptoms.

Press the point between your partner's neck and shoulder to relieve shoulder pain.

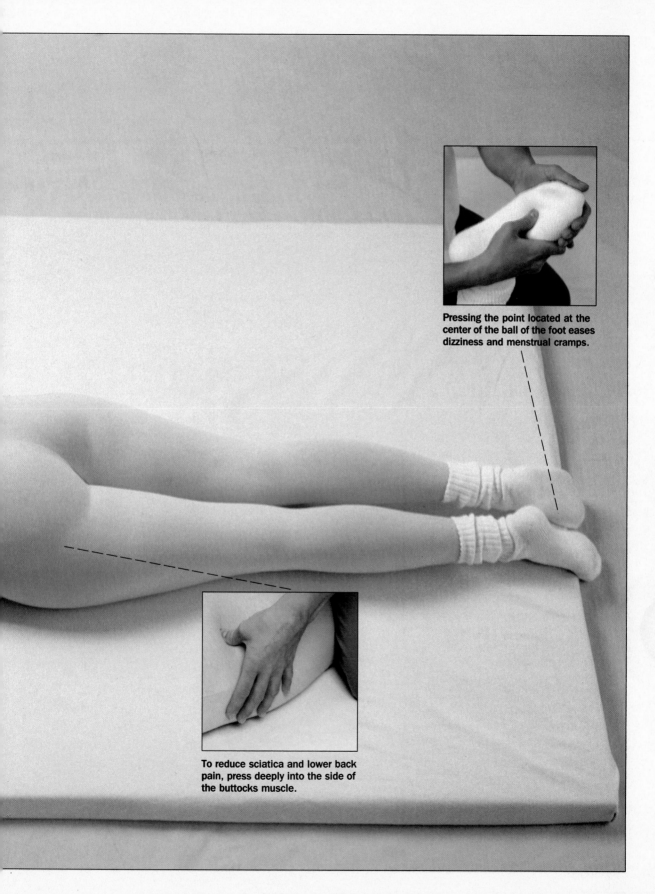

Pressing the point located at the center of the ball of the foot eases dizziness and menstrual cramps.

To reduce sciatica and lower back pain, press deeply into the side of the buttocks muscle.

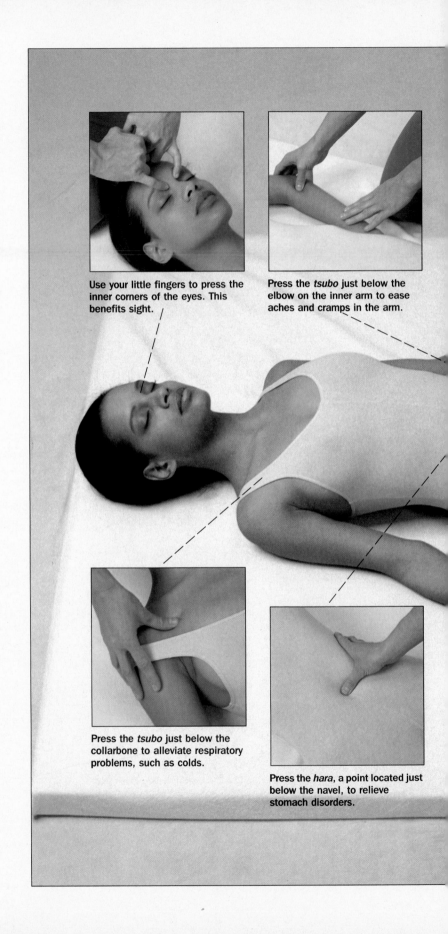

Use your little fingers to press the inner corners of the eyes. This benefits sight.

Press the *tsubo* just below the elbow on the inner arm to ease aches and cramps in the arm.

Press the *tsubo* just below the collarbone to alleviate respiratory problems, such as colds.

Press the *hara*, a point located just below the navel, to relieve stomach disorders.

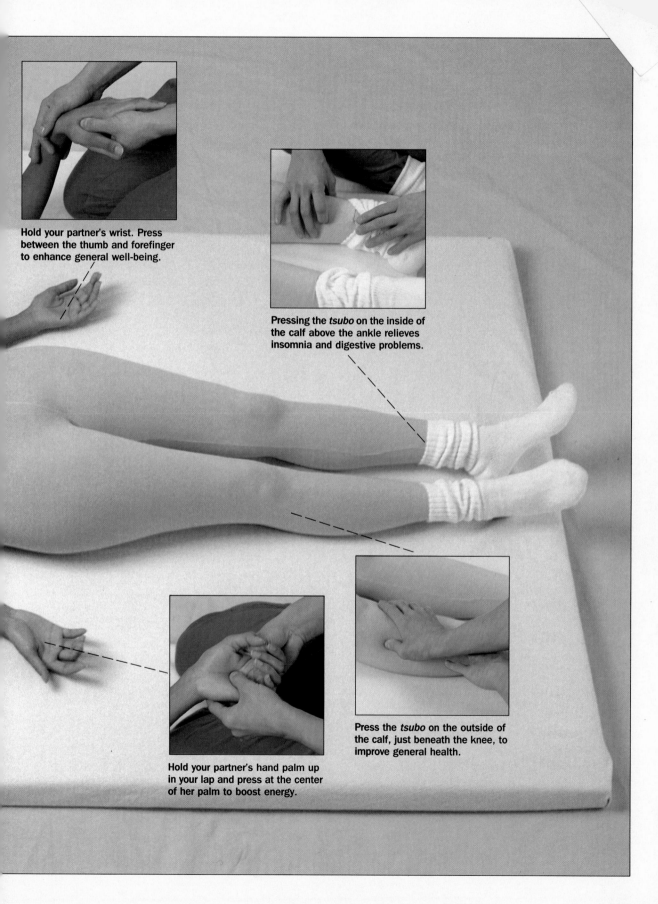

Hold your partner's wrist. Press between the thumb and forefinger to enhance general well-being.

Pressing the *tsubo* on the inside of the calf above the ankle relieves insomnia and digestive problems.

Hold your partner's hand palm up in your lap and press at the center of her palm to boost energy.

Press the *tsubo* on the outside of the calf, just beneath the knee, to improve general health.

Reflexology

Like shiatsu, reflexology is a pressure-point therapy that works very specific points. But instead of *tsubos*, you press reflex points in the feet. Like all Eastern massage methods, reflexology is based on an energy that circulates throughout the body, which reflexologists believe terminates in the feet. It is here that the energy can pool or become trapped, so working the feet will release the energy and restore the body. (As with shiatsu, this theory of energy circulation has yet to be proved experimentally.)

Each reflex in the foot corresponds closely to a part of the body, as shown in the reflexology chart below. The toes correspond to the head and neck; the heels, to the lower back and pelvic area. In between lie the internal organs. Working these reflexes will relieve tension in associated body areas: For example, when you press the balls of the toes, you are affecting the sinuses.

The four basic finger and thumb techniques used in reflexology are demonstrated on the opposite page; the treatment sequence is on the following two pages. Thumb walking and finger walking — creeping, caterpillar-like movements — are the most frequently used techniques. Work on very specific reflexes requires two other techniques, rotation on a point and hook and back-up.

To achieve adequate leverage for these techniques, you need to hold the foot correctly. When working with your right hand, wrap your left hand around the toes to hold them straight and keep the heel steady. Reverse the hold when you work with your left hand.

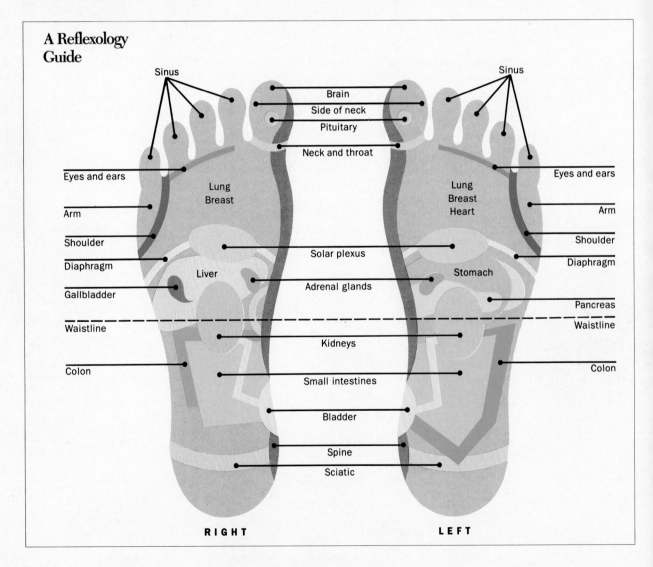

A Reflexology Guide

Sinus — Sinus

Brain
Side of neck
Pituitary
Neck and throat

Eyes and ears — Eyes and ears

Lung Breast — Lung Breast Heart

Arm — Arm

Shoulder — Shoulder

Diaphragm — Diaphragm

Solar plexus

Liver — Stomach

Adrenal glands

Gallbladder

Pancreas

Waistline — Waistline

Kidneys

Colon — Colon

Small intestines

Bladder

Spine

Sciatic

RIGHT **LEFT**

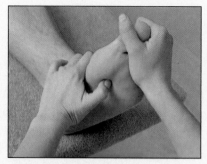

THUMB WALKING Press the outside of your thumb into the sole. Inch forward by bending and unbending the thumb.

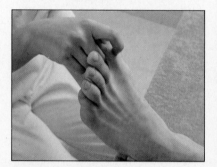

FINGER WALKING Inch forward with your index finger by bending and unbending the first joint.

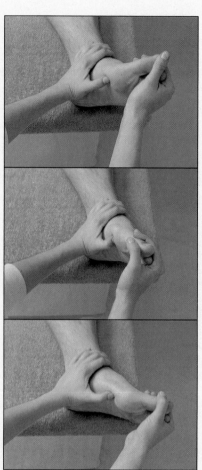

ROTATION ON A POINT Press just beneath the ball of the foot with your thumb *(top)*. With your other hand around the toes, pull the foot toward you *(center)* and then around *(above)*.

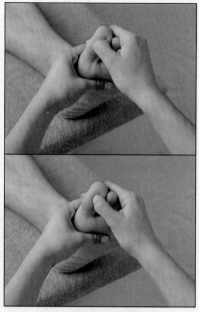

HOOK AND BACK-UP Where the skin is tough, press firmly with your thumb *(top)* and push the skin back *(above)*.

A Reflexology Sequence

One advantage of reflexology is its convenience — your partner only needs to remove his shoes and socks. Your partner should be positioned so that his feet are slightly above your lap. Ideally, he should be lying on a table or seated in a reclining chair to give his foot support from below and to give you maximum leverage.

Treat one foot, then the other. Use the diagram on page 76 to incorporate any additional reflexes you feel would benefit your partner. If you are uncertain about the location of a particular reflex, you can be sure you have covered it if you thoroughly thumb walk up each zone.

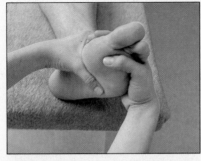

1. Squeeze, wring and rub your partner's feet to relax them and prepare them for deeper work.

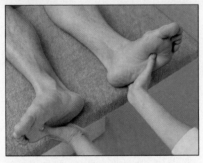

2. Place your thumbs at the center of each foot, just below the ball, to treat the solar plexus. Press for 10 seconds.

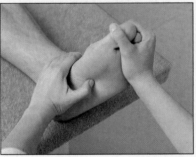

3. Thumb walk from the heel to the base of each toe. Walk up five times, working in line with each toe.

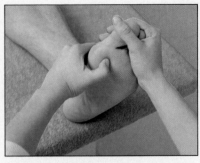

4. Thumb walk across the entire ball of the foot, an area that corresponds to the chest and the lungs.

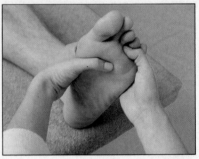

5. Use the inside surface of your thumb to walk across the neck reflexes, located between the toes and the ball of the foot.

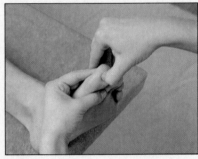

6. Thumb walk down the inside of the big toe, then finger walk down the outside. Repeat this on each toe to work the head reflexes.

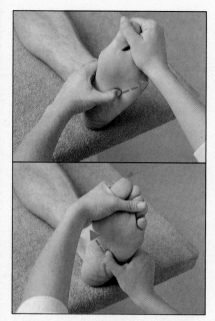

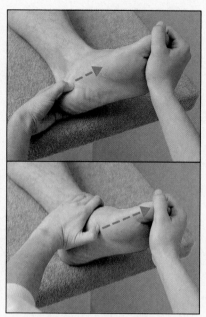

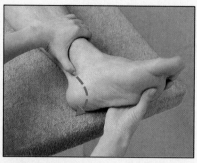

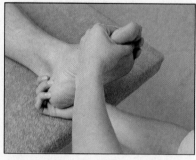

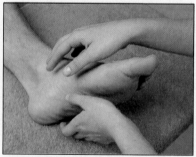

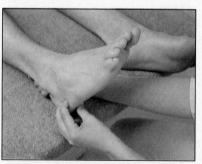

7. Thumb walk diagonally across the reflexes of the internal organs at the center of the foot. Work from the inside to the outside *(top)*, then from the outside to the inside *(above)*.

8. Cup the heel and thumb walk along the inside of the foot from the heel to the ankle *(top)*. Then grasp the ankle and continue thumb walking to the big toe *(above)*. This benefits reflexes for the spine.

9. Finger walk along the area corresponding to the hip and knee, located beneath the ankle on the outside of the foot.

10. Hold your partner's foot above the ankle and thumb walk down to the heel to relieve conditions such as sciatica.

11. With your middle finger, rotate the reflex for the sexual organs, located halfway between your anklebone and heel.

12. Conclude the reflexology sequence by holding the solar plexus, then passing your fingers lightly over the entire foot.

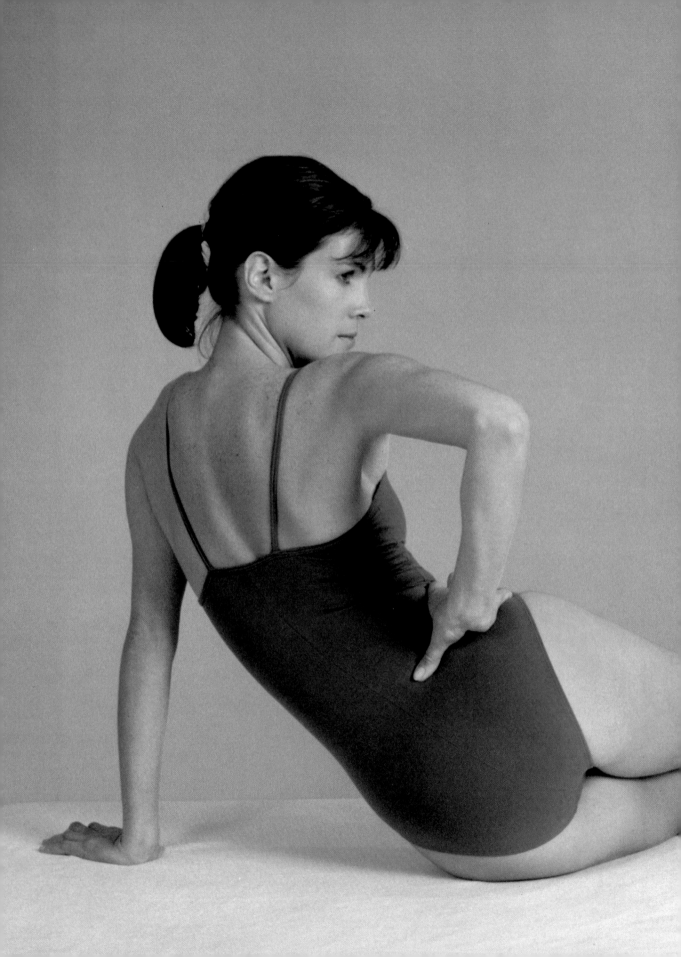

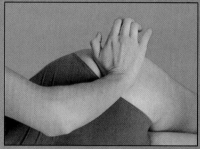

Kneel and place your fists next to your spine. Use your knuckles to effleurage up and down your back.

Lie on your side and circular-palm petrissage down your buttocks. Cover the side, then roll to your other side and repeat.

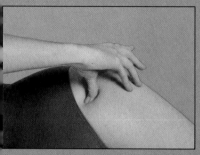
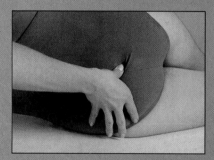

Use your thumb to press the *tsubo* located at the center of the outside of your buttocks. Repeat on your other side.

Use your thumb for circular kneading on the sacrum, or tailbone, located at the base of the spine.

Self-Massage/1

I f you do not have a partner to work with, it is possible to perform massage on yourself, although self-massage does have some shortcomings. Most obviously, you cannot reach all the areas of your body that a partner can reach. And even on some areas that you can reach, you will find it difficult or impossible to apply a stroke with the proper leverage or pressure. More important, since some of your muscles must work to perform the stroke, you cannot fully relax your body.

Although these shortcomings make it more superficial than a partner massage, self-massage can still relieve muscle tension and help you to relax. And it has a unique benefit: As you directly experience the effects of performing a massage, you learn what feels good and what does not — knowledge that will help you give a better massage to a partner.

Specific, localized strokes, such as pressure and friction, are the mainstay of self-massage. These strokes tend to be more effective than broader strokes such as effleurage, since it is easier to get the proper leverage — especially on the upper body. Because they are pressure-based routines, self-shiatsu and self-reflexology are particuarly effective. Do not use oil when doing pressure techniques, since it may cause your hands to slip.

The techniques shown here and on the following 10 pages include Swedish, shiatsu and reflexology techniques. A final section on cosmetic massage presents a complete routine that can improve facial circulation.

Sit on the floor with your legs extended and your left arm supporting you. Reach behind with your right hand and use your thumb to exert pressure next to your spine. Work up and down the lower back. Switch sides and repeat on the other side of the spine with your left hand.

Self-Massage/2

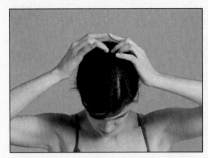

For tension and headache relief, use your middle fingers to press the *tsubo* located at the center of the crown.

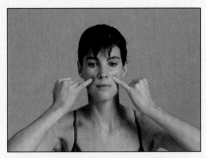

With your little fingers, press the *tsubos* that are located about an inch from the sides of your nose.

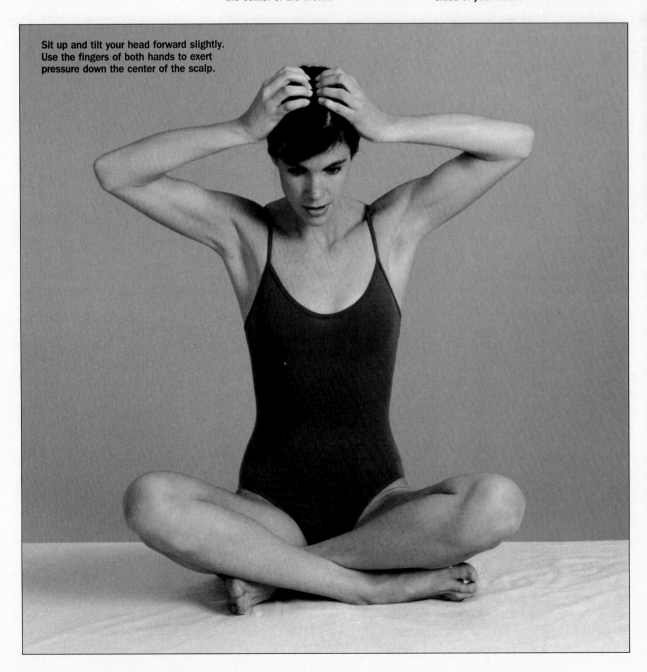

Sit up and tilt your head forward slightly. Use the fingers of both hands to exert pressure down the center of the scalp.

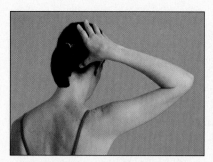

Clasp your fingers around your head for support and use your thumb to press along the ridge between your skull and neck.

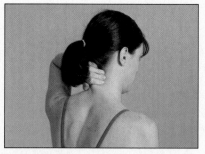

Grasp the muscles at the back of your neck and squeeze them between your fingers and palm. Do not press on the spine.

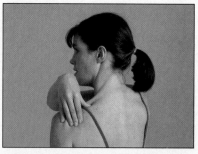

Reach over one shoulder to press the *tsubo* located in the middle of the shoulder. Repeat on the other shoulder.

Squeeze the muscle running down the sides of your neck and across your shoulder. Repeat on the other side.

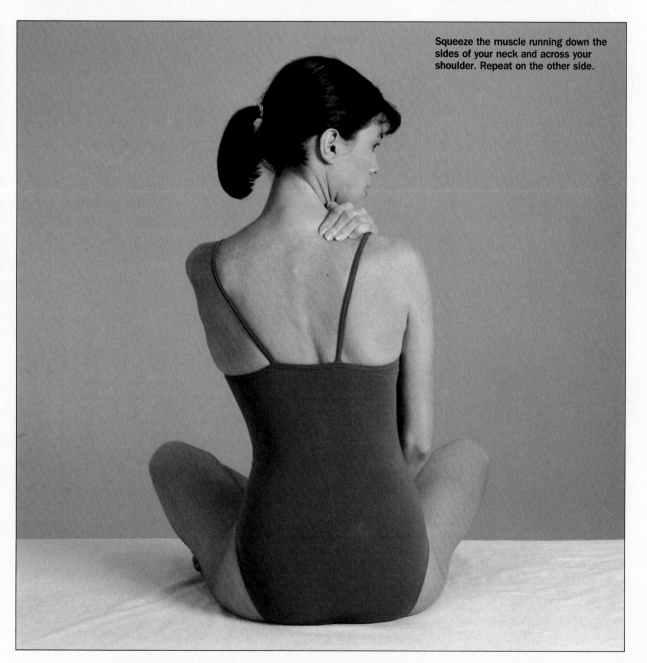

Self-Massage/3

Lie on your back with your knees bent.
Place one hand over the other and use your
fingertips to effleurage clockwise around
your abdomen, starting from the lower right
corner. Repeat twice.

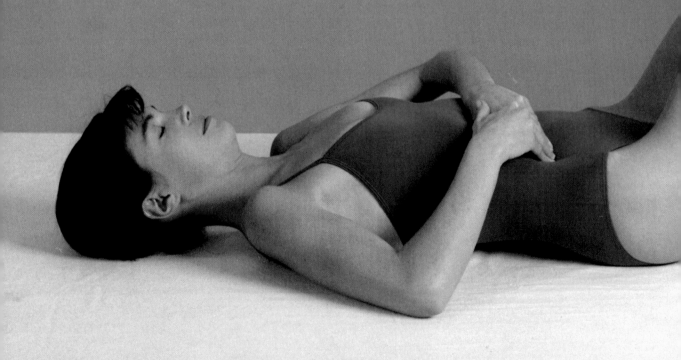

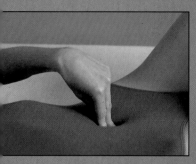

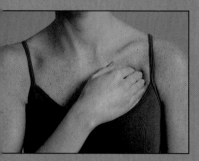

ress the *hara*, located about one and a
alf inches below your navel. Hold for about
0 seconds.

t up and use your fingertips for circular
iction around your chest. Women should
void putting pressure on their breasts.

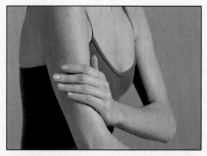

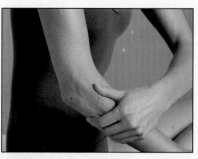

Use broad, flat-hand effleurage to stroke
from your wrist up to your shoulder. Glide
back and repeat twice.

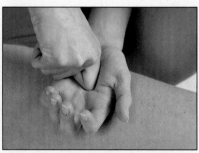

Place your hand in your lap and press the
center of your palm with the joint of your
forefinger; hold for 10 seconds.

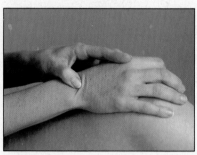

Bend your arm and support it in your lap.
Grasp your forearm and use your thumb for
circular friction at the elbow.

Turn one palm down and use your thumb for
transverse friction across your wrist. Repeat
the sequence on the other arm.

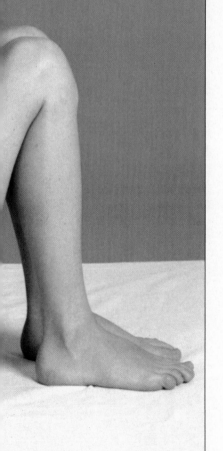

Self-Massage/4

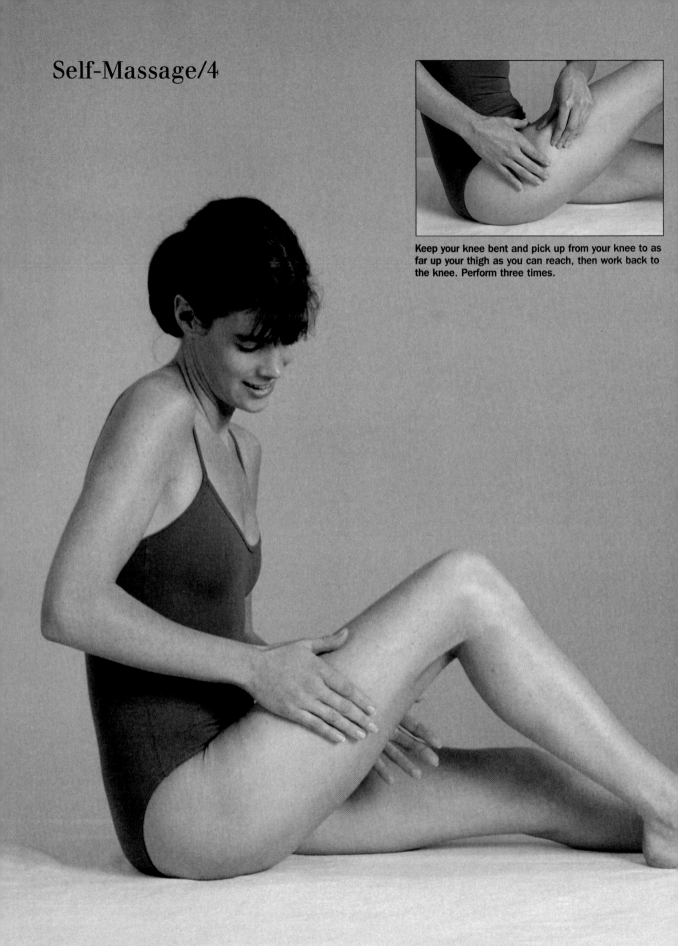

Keep your knee bent and pick up from your knee to as far up your thigh as you can reach, then work back to the knee. Perform three times.

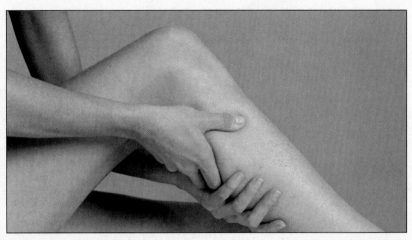

Support your right calf with your left hand to give you leverage. Grasping the calf with your right hand, use your thumb to press the *tsubo* just below the knee on the outside of the calf.

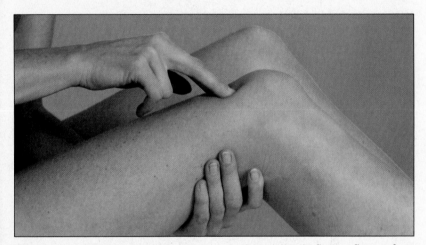

Hold your right thigh just under the knee with your left hand. Use the first two fingers of your right hand for circular friction around your knee; then do circular friction around your ankle. Repeat the entire routine on your left leg.

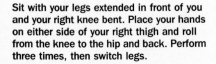

Sit with your legs extended in front of you and your right knee bent. Place your hands on either side of your right thigh and roll from the knee to the hip and back. Perform three times, then switch legs.

Self-Reflexology

One of the most effective forms of self-massage is self-reflexology. Because the feet are so easy to reach, you will be able to give yourself a full session that provides many of the benefits of reflexology with a partner. And, as with all self-massage, it provides you with the opportunity for practice, so you can discover firsthand which techniques feel best.

For self-reflexology, you should sit either cross-legged, as shown at right, or with one leg extended straight in front of you, bracing the foot on which you are working, as shown on the opposite page. To begin the basic sequence shown here, relax your foot by squeezing and wringing it. Refer back to the diagram on page 76 if you wish to incorporate any additional reflexes.

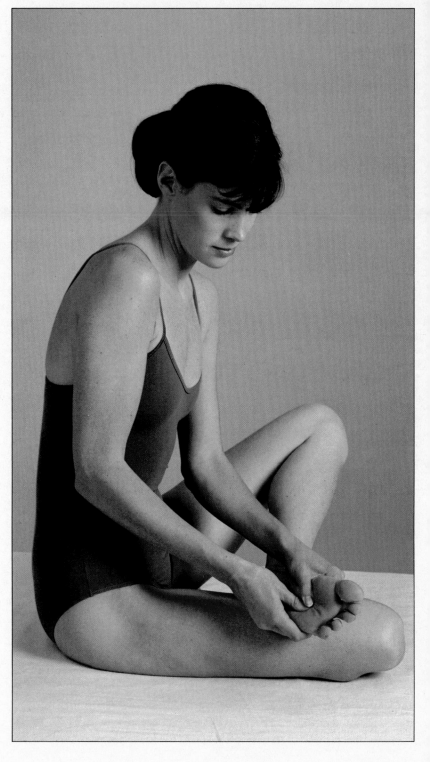

Press the solar plexus reflex, just below the center of the ball of the foot, with both thumbs. Hold for eight to 10 seconds.

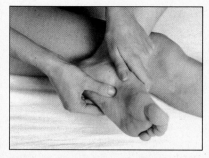

Thumb walk the five zones of the foot that run down from each toe.

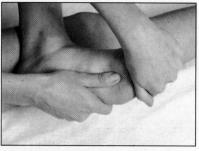

Do rotations across the diaphragm line running just under the ball of the foot.

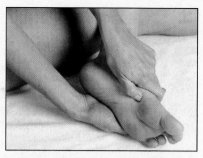

Locate the adrenal reflex, near the inside of the ball of the foot, and do a rotation.

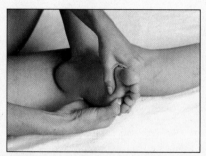

Thumb walk the ridge between the toes and foot, which corresponds to the neck.

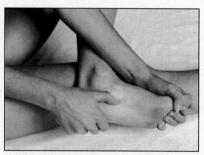

Thumb walk up the inside edge of the foot, from the heel to the toes, to work the spine.

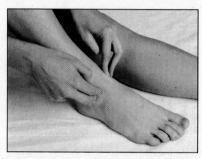

Finger walk the top and sides of the ankle along the reflexes for the sexual organs.

Cosmetic Massage/1

A facial massage cannot eliminate lines or wrinkles, but its circulatory effects can benefit the skin's tone and appearance. Connective tissue in the face can trap blood and lymph, which carry oxygen and other nutrients to and from the tissues. When this occurs, decreased oxygenation may impair the health of tissues and adversely affect skin color and tone.

Clinical studies have repeatedly shown that the strokes of massage increase circulation and tissue oxygenation, thus improving the appearance of the skin. Furthermore, simply relaxing the muscles in your face will decrease tension, a major cause of wrinkles.

Thoroughly cleanse your face and apply a light moisturizer before beginning the sequence shown here. You might want to practice these techniques in front of a mirror to familiarize yourself with them.

Cosmetic massage can also be incorporated into partner massage. If you wear contact lenses, be sure to remove them before having a facial massage.

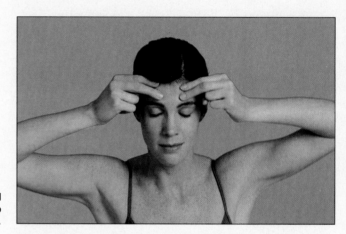

Start at the center of your forehead and use the first two fingers of both hands to stroke upward. Work outward.

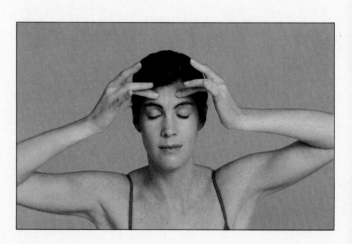

Start at your eyebrows and use your middle finger for circular friction across the forehead. Work toward your hairline.

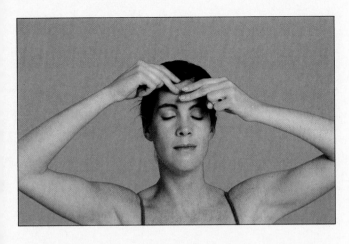

Use the first two fingers of both hands to stroke diagonally across the forehead. Start at one side and work across.

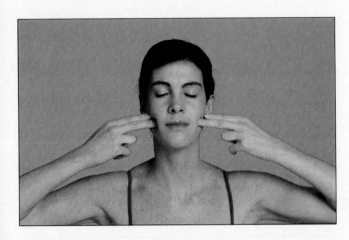

Start at the center of your chin and use the first two fingers of both hands for circular friction. Work upward to your ears.

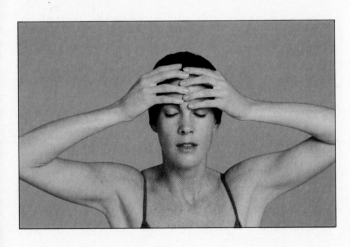

Bring your fingers together over the center of your forehead. Exert light pressure as you slide them apart toward your temples.

Cosmetic Massage/2

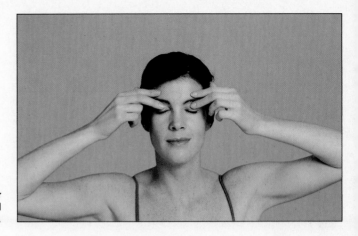

Place your two middle fingers at the inner corners of your eyes. Stroke around and underneath the eyes.

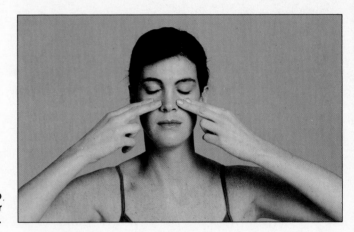

Stroke down your nose with the first two fingers of both hands, then use circular friction across the cheekbones.

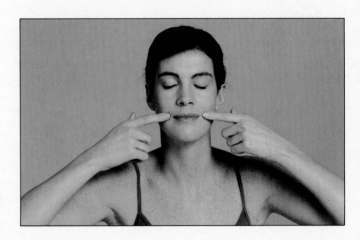

Start just beneath your nose and use your index finger to stroke around your mouth. Return and repeat.

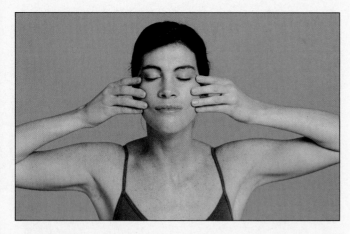

Place your slighty separated fingers on either side of your nose. Maintain even pressure as you stroke toward your hairline.

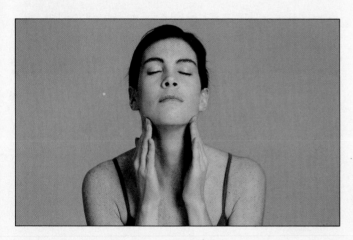

Use your first fingers for circular friction along the jawline, from the ears to the center of the chin. Repeat at mouth level.

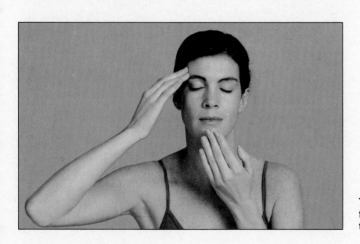

Tap lightly over the entire face, using the first two fingers of both hands. Avoid tapping directly on the eyes.

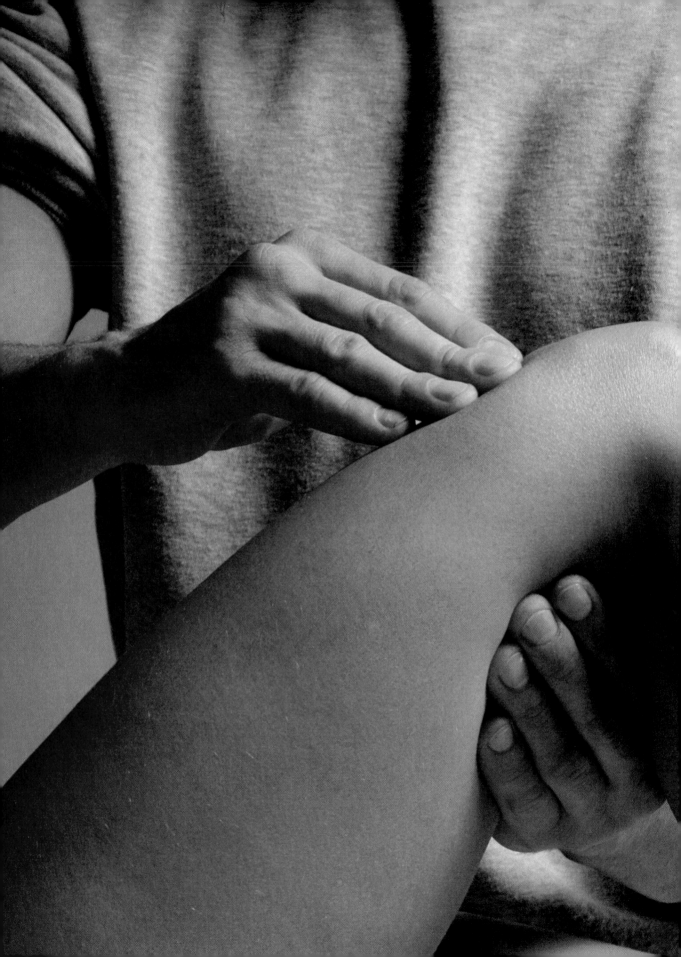

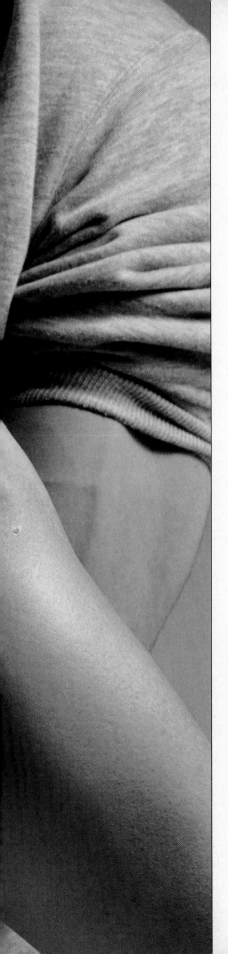

CHAPTER FOUR

Sports Massage

*Deep strokes for soothing and
invigorating muscles before
or after a workout*

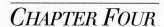

Anyone who exercises regularly, whether a relative beginner or a longtime fitness practitioner, can benefit from sports massage. Its aims are specific: preventing injury and enhancing flexibility. As in full-body massage, relaxation is one of the benefits. But the strokes of sports massage, derived from Swedish massage and trigger-point pressure techniques, are unique in that they place particular emphasis on reaching deeply into the musculature. Also, sports massage focuses on muscle groups used in a specific exercise. If your partner is a swimmer, for example, much of your massage work will concentrate on his or her upper body.

The causes of soreness range from a build-up of metabolic by-products like lactic acid to the development of microtears, scars and adhesions in the muscles and surrounding tissues. In addition, very tense or tight muscles can increase the risk of injury during workouts. This chapter concentrates on preventive massage techniques that will reduce the potential for injury. Used regularly, sports-massage

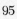

95

routines will not only help keep your muscles flexible, but also stimulate circulation, increase lymphatic flow and aid in clearing lactic acid from your muscles. If you have any sudden or chronic pain, or suspect injury, consult your physician before having a massage. Only a licensed massage therapist or physical therapist should massage injured tissue.

Some of the injury-prevention techniques shown here can also be used immediately before or after a workout or competition. Massaging those muscles likely to be affected by a long run or bike ride, for example, will loosen them. Likewise, a massage after exercising helps cut down recovery time — in fact, one study found that including massage with the usual rest period tripled the subjects' work capacity. Several studies have also demonstrated that a postworkout massage brings the pulse rate back to normal faster and hastens the recovery of muscle efficiency. Many athletes report that regular sports massage eases stiffness or soreness, thus enabling them to shorten the intervals between workouts.

Certain sports-massage techniques have been used to treat athletic injuries. But only a licensed massage therapist, physical therapist or athletic trainer should work with injured tissue. And any injury sustained through participation in sports or exercise should first be diagnosed by a physician.

Three movements account for a majority of the work done in preventive sports massage. Deep stroking, performed by moving the thumbs lengthwise up the muscle, forces large amounts of blood to circulate and eliminates metabolic by-products. Broad cross-fiber strokes, in which your thumbs cross the muscle at a 90-degree angle, separate muscle fibers from each other to break adhesions, which can diminish power and pliability. Compressions — rhythmic pumping executed primarily by the palm of the hand — press muscle against bone and spread out individual fibers. Compressions are a mainstay of a preworkout massage because they produce a durable hyperemia, an increase in the supplies of blood and oxygen available to fuel the muscles during exercise.

There are several more specialized techniques in sports massage. Local cross-fiber stroking is used on tendons and ligaments to make muscle and connective tissue more pliable. Jostling relaxes the entire muscle by gently squeezing and shaking it; you can incorporate it into a massage whenever the muscles you are working on become tense. Finally, pressure techniques are used to locate the body's trigger points — small areas of deep tenderness within a muscle — and then relax them.

The following 26 pages demonstrate how to apply these techniques to the muscle groups illustrated opposite. When performing a sports massage, proceed slowly to ensure that you cover a muscle completely. For example, in broad cross-fiber stroking, you should move forward at thumb-length intervals, using even pressure. Likewise, when deep stroking, work up the entire length of the muscle, then move over one inch and repeat the technique, continuing until you have

Musculature

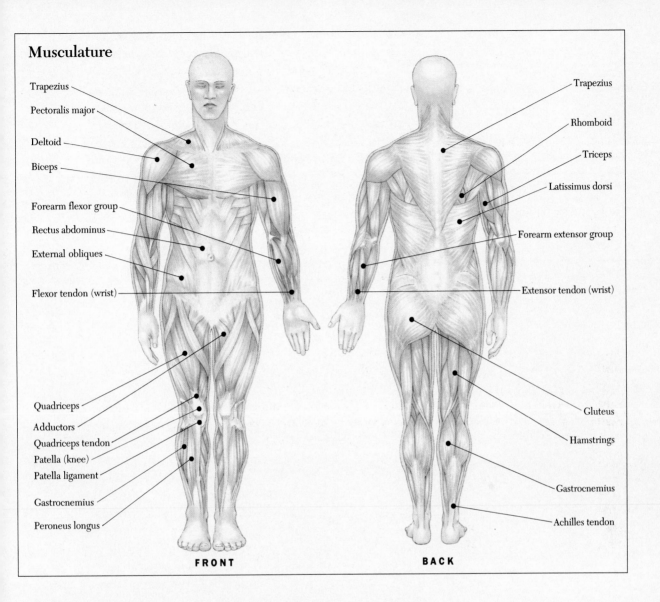

Trapezius
Pectoralis major
Deltoid
Biceps
Forearm flexor group
Rectus abdominus
External obliques
Flexor tendon (wrist)
Quadriceps
Adductors
Quadriceps tendon
Patella (knee)
Patella ligament
Gastrocnemius
Peroneus longus

Trapezius
Rhomboid
Triceps
Latissimus dorsi
Forearm extensor group
Extensor tendon (wrist)
Gluteus
Hamstrings
Gastrocnemius
Achilles tendon

FRONT

BACK

encircled the whole muscle to reach as many fibers as possible. (Use broad cross-fiber and deep stroking only on the bulky part of the muscle, not at the narrow muscle ends, where heavy longitudinal strokes can damage tendons and ligaments.)

Perform these massage routines symmetrically, so that you work both sides of the body identically. Also, work each body part completely before moving on to the next. For example, finish massaging one leg before you switch to the other leg. Always pay attention to your partner's pain threshold to determine how much pressure you can comfortably apply.

Do not use oil for trigger-point techniques, which work into a small area; oil may cause your hands to slip. Likewise, avoid oil in a pre-event massage, since it might clog pores and prevent perspiration. Otherwise, you should use oil in sports massage just as you would with a full-body massage.

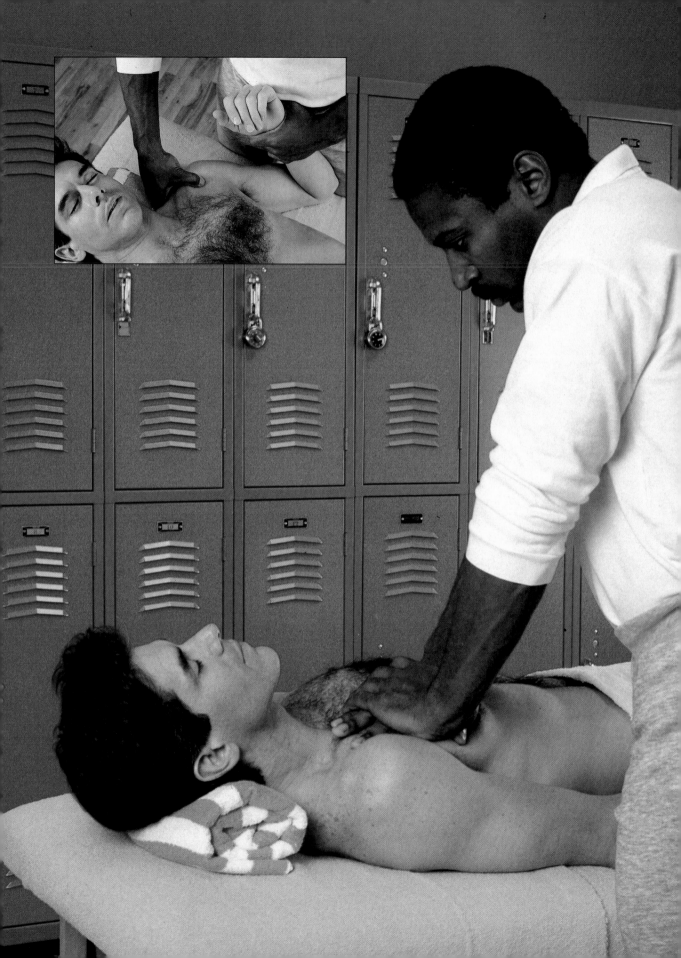

Chest

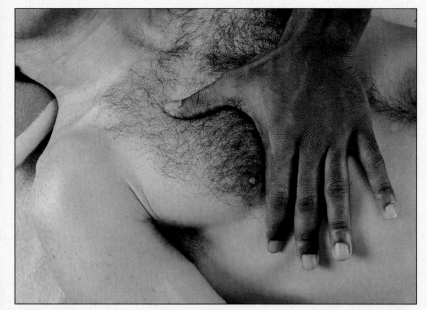

BROAD CROSS-FIBER Spread your hand so that your thumb points toward your partner's shoulder. Start near the shoulder and roll outward. Repeat at thumb-length intervals, working down your partner's chest.

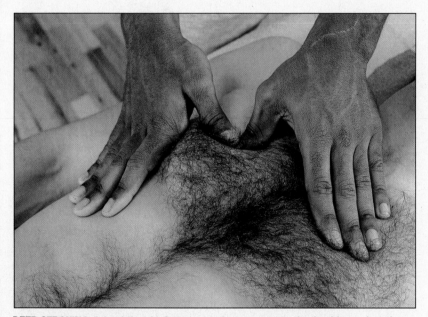

DEEP STROKING (joined-thumb) Start just below your partner's shoulder and stroke diagonally across his chest to the midline. Repeat the strokes at one-inch intervals along the chest to cover the entire muscle.

COMPRESSIONS Cover your partner's entire chest with hand-on-hand compressions *(opposite)*, avoiding the ribs. Then bend one arm at the elbow *(inset)* to locate the tendons that attach it to the torso. Clamp your hand around your partner's shoulder and apply a one-thumb local cross-fiber stroke. Repeat on the other arm.

The complex musculature of the chest, which attaches to both the shoulders and the ribs, affects arm movements, especially those of the shoulder. For example, chest muscles are integral to performing a basic push-up. Participants in any sport that uses the arms, particularly body builders and weight lifters, will benefit from the massage techniques shown below.

Most chest massage will work the large, triangular pectoralis major muscles, which are located on either side of the chest and cover the deeper musculature. The fibers of the pectorals run diagonally across the chest from the shoulder. Keep this direction in mind when you massage the area — especially when you use broad cross-fiber strokes, the effectiveness of which depends on stroking perpendicular to the grain of the muscle.

When performing the following massage strokes on women, work around the breasts, avoiding any direct pressure on them.

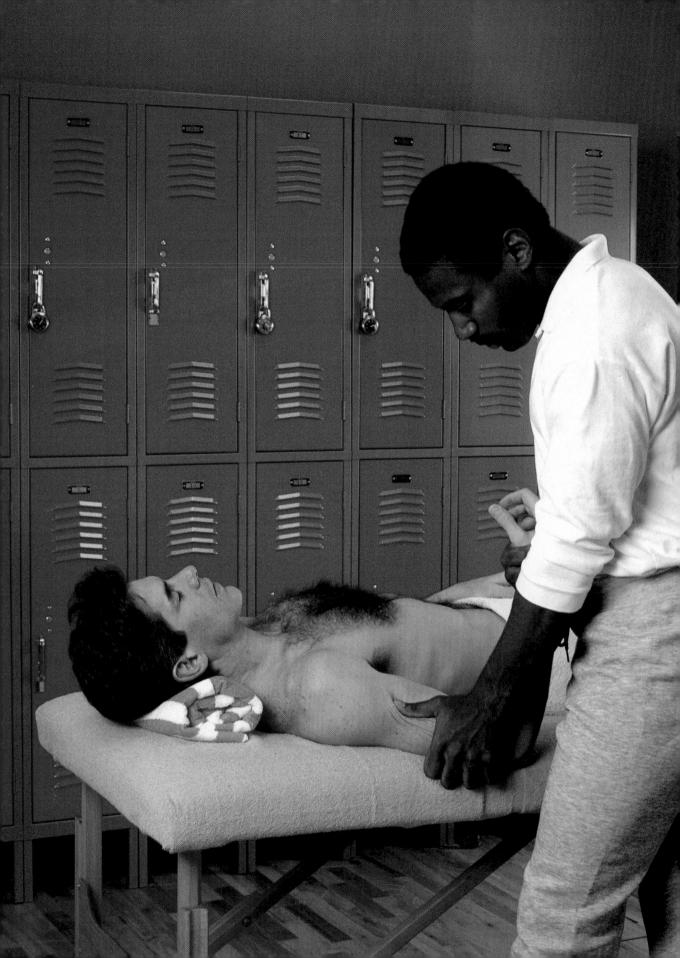

Upper Arms

Anyone who plays baseball, basketball, golf or any racquet sport will benefit from an upper arm massage. There are two major muscles in the upper arm: the biceps, located on the front of the arm just below the shoulder, and the triceps, on the back of the arm. These muscles complement each other; the biceps flex the arm and the triceps extend it.

Strokes to the biceps are demonstrated here; the same movements can be applied to the triceps when your partner is lying on his or her stomach.

The biceps and triceps are attached to the forearm by tendons that extend to a few inches below the elbow. Local cross-fiber strokes, not shown here, should be applied to these easily irritated tendons. Avoid direct pressure on the elbow.

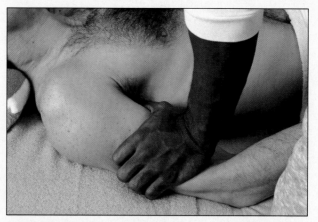

COMPRESSIONS (one-hand) Bend your partner's elbow; hold his forearm in your right hand. Grasp his arm with your left hand and apply compressions with your palm on the belly of the muscle.

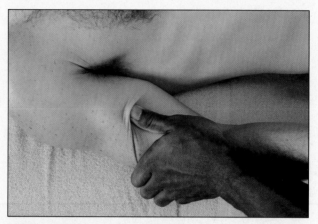

DEEP STROKING (one-thumb) Place your right hand under your partner's upper left arm for leverage. Stroke up the biceps with your left thumb and glide back. Repeat at one-inch intervals.

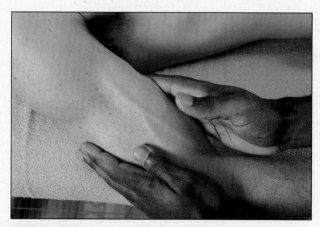

BROAD CROSS-FIBER Bend your partner's right arm at the elbow. With your left hand, grasp his arm a few inches above the elbow with your thumb pointing toward his armpit *(opposite)*. Roll out. Work upward on the biceps to the shoulder; then change hands and apply broad cross-fiber strokes to the inside of the arm.

JOSTLING With your partner's arm lying flat, grasp his biceps with both hands. Rhythmically shake the muscle, working up toward his armpit and back down.

Forearm

The forearm has two major muscle groups, each containing numerous small muscles: The flexor group allows the wrist to bend; the extensor group straightens it out. These muscles attach to tendons that occupy much of the lower forearm.

Because of the number of tendons in the forearm, you should perform many local cross-fiber strokes on this area. Any tendons encased in a sheath, such as those of the wrist and ankle, must be massaged as they are stretched. So bend the wrist while massaging to keep the tendons flexed.

When you perform broad cross-fiber massage on the forearm, you will notice an unevenness, due to the number of different muscles and tendons in this relatively small area. This will create a plucking sensation as you cross the forearm muscles.

LOCAL CROSS-FIBER Rest your partner's bent right arm on your leg. Hold his right hand in yours for stability. Grasp his elbow with your left hand, and move your thumb back and forth at the tendons.

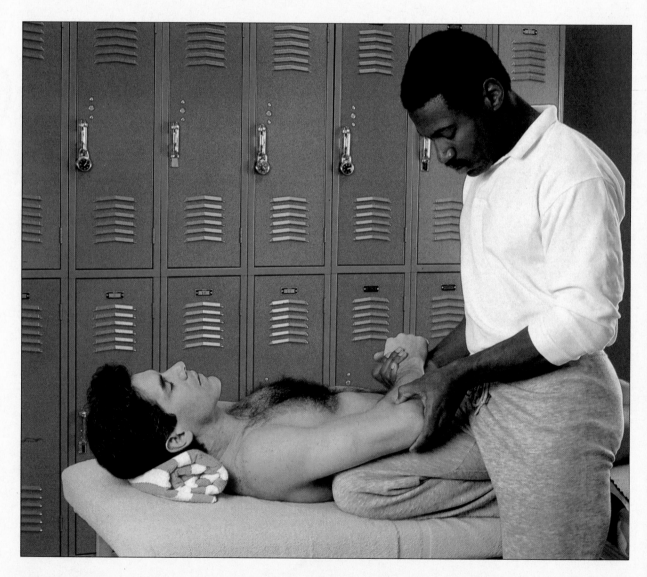

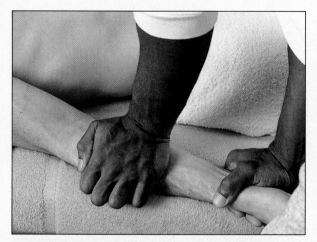

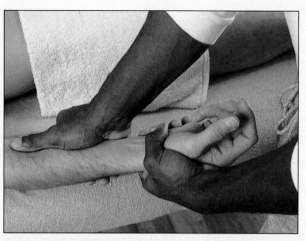

COMPRESSIONS Place your partner's right arm palm up and hold it above the wrist with your right hand. Use the palm of your left hand to cover the upper forearm with compressions.

BROAD CROSS-FIBER Use your right hand for broad cross-fiber on the upper forearm, working up to the elbow. Turn his arm over and work the outside of the forearm.

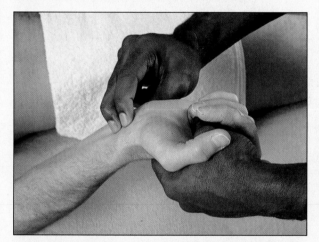

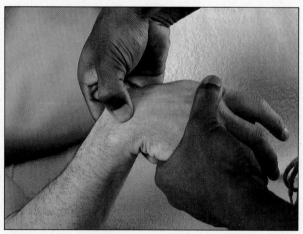

LOCAL CROSS-FIBER (to inner wrist) Hold your partner's hand and bend the wrist back. Use two fingers and stroke rapidly back and forth across the tendon between the hand and forearm.

LOCAL CROSS-FIBER (to outer wrist) Turn your partner's hand over and bend it forward. Grasp around the wrist with your right hand and use your thumb to stroke across the tendon.

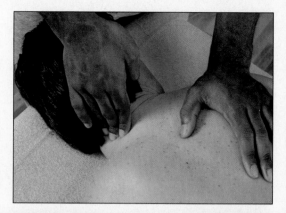

LOCAL CROSS-FIBER (to base of neck)
Starting at the base of the skull on the right side, work next to the spine with two fingers. Continue to the base of the neck.

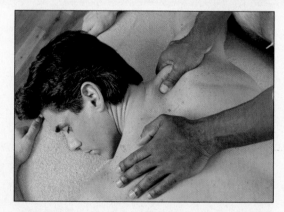

BROAD CROSS-FIBER (to trapezius) Bend your partner's arm up and turn his head away. Grasp his right shoulder and work from his shoulder into his neck.

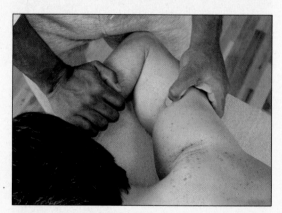

LOCAL CROSS-FIBER (to deltoid) Bend your partner's right arm over his head. Grasp his arm at the base of the deltoid with your left hand and work across with your thumb.

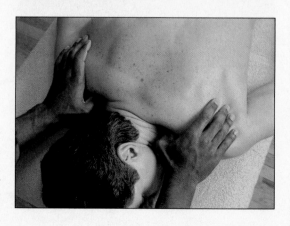

TRIGGER POINTS Stand at your partner's head and search with your thumbs for trigger points clustered together along the top of the trapezius.

Neck and Shoulders

Because of its intricate musculature and its constant use in almost all daily activities, the neck is a prime target for tension. It is also integrally involved with body alignment, since the top seven vertebrae of the spine are located there.

While the neck is not actually the focus of most sports, except for some weight-lifting routines, the muscular stresses of sports and exercise indirectly affect it. For example, a tennis serve places uneven pressure on your body; the muscles of the neck compensate for this imbalance, thus bearing the stress themselves.

The shoulder muscles operate in conjunction with those of the neck, and are important for supporting the neck, as well as for providing power in activities like racquet sports that require strength or agility. The trapezius, which runs along the top of the shoulders and functions in conjunction with the deltoids (one of the major muscles of the shoulder), is a frequent site of neck-related trigger points.

Because there are so many bones in the neck, massage in this area can be painful. Work gently, avoiding compression techniques.

JOSTLING (deltoids) Bend your partner's arm to relax it. Grasp the deltoid with one hand and shake it, working up the muscle to the shoulder and back down.

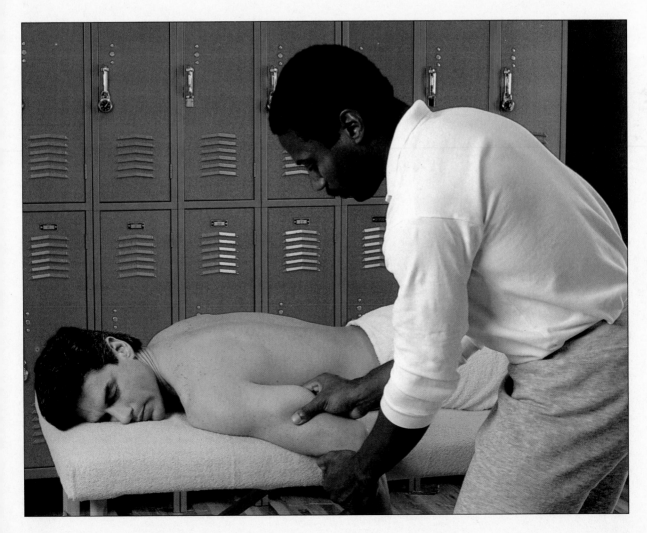

Upper Back

A strong, healthy back is a prerequisite for most forms of exercise and sports. Unfortunately, with its elaborate musculature, the back is easily injured. Massage will help keep your partner's back in optimal condition. During a back massage, pay particular attention to any knots you locate while performing either local or broad cross-fiber strokes. Repeated treatments of these vulnerable areas will help prevent serious muscular problems that could interfere with athletic performance.

The upper-back muscles, in addition to controlling back movement, are important for arm strength. These muscles, which are smaller than those of the lower back, crisscross in so many directions that smooth, broad massage movements are not easy to execute. If you have difficulty with the broad cross-fiber shown here, concentrate on the trigger points. Techniques that focus on the upper back are presented on these two pages; lower back techniques follow on the next two pages. Treat the upper and lower back as a whole for massage purposes.

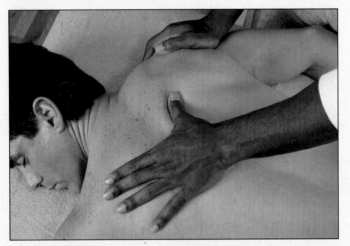

COMPRESSIONS (hand-on-hand) Pump rapidly over the upper back, doing about 40 compressions in all. Avoid the spine.

BROAD CROSS-FIBER (to trapezius) Work the muscle that runs right along the shoulder blade, but avoid the bone.

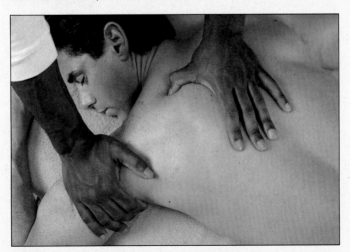

TRIGGER POINTS Search for trigger points along the top of the shoulder blade, working outward from the middle of the back.

BROAD CROSS-FIBER (to rhomboids) Bend your partner's right arm behind his back and use the palm of your right hand to lift his shoulder *(opposite)*. Use your left thumb for broad cross-fiber stroking underneath the shoulder blade. Repeat on the other side of the back.

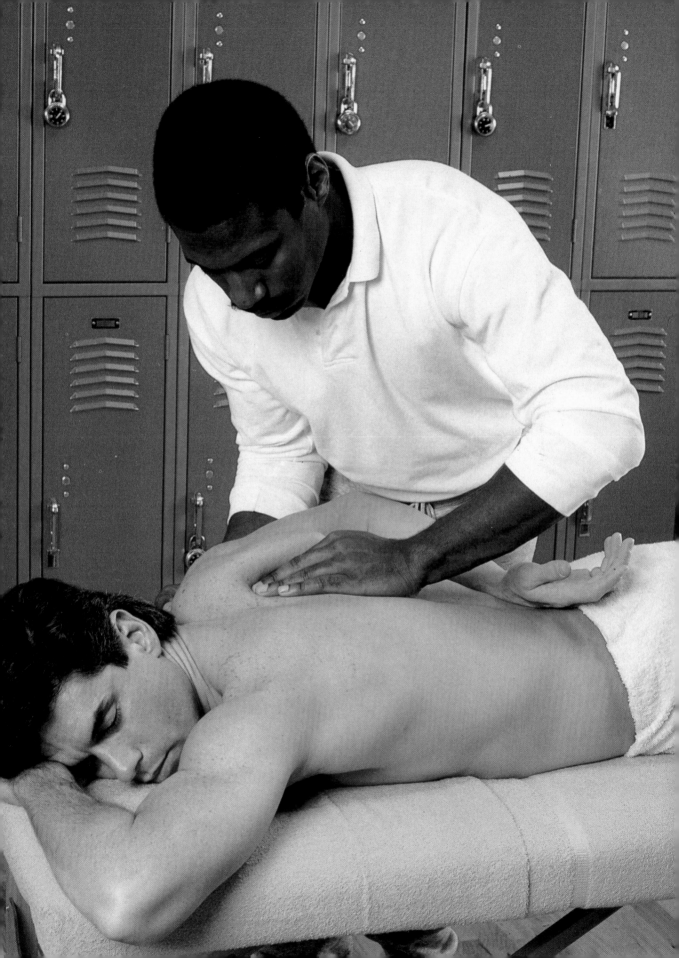

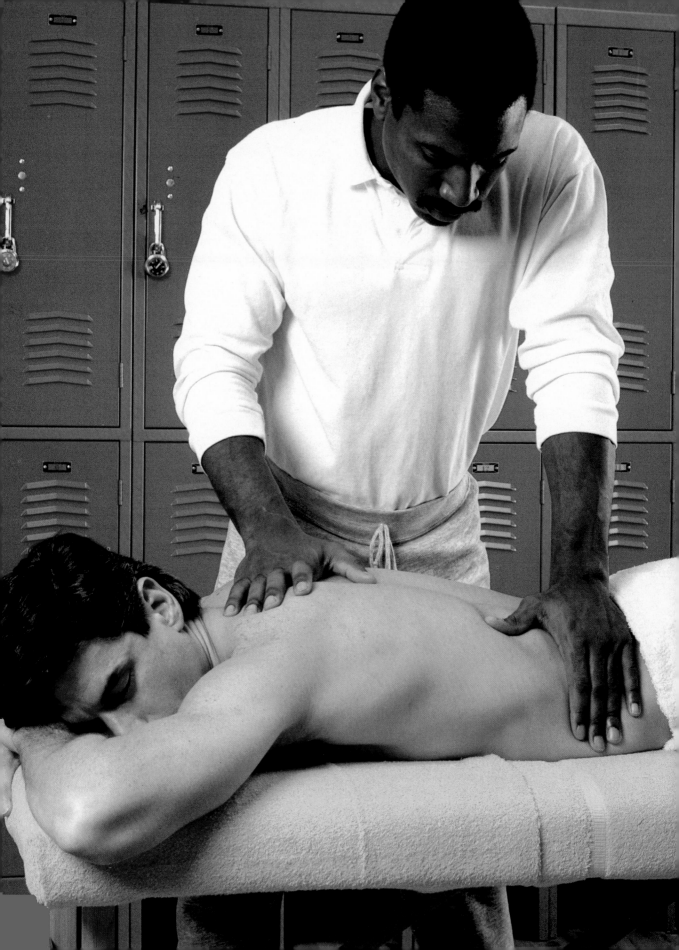

Lower Back

Whether or not you are an athlete, you probably have experienced back pain. A recent study found that fully 80 percent of the American population suffers from back pain during their lifetime. Most of this pain occurs in the lower back. While any sport is likely to put additional strain on the lower back, cyclists, skiers and golfers are among those most at risk, due to the amount of bending these activities require.

The major muscles of the lower back are the spinal erectors, which are narrow, barrel-shaped muscles running the full length of the spine, and the latissimus dorsi, which runs diagonally from just below the waist to under the armpit on each side of the body. In general, the lower back muscles are either long or broad, so you will be able to use smooth, deep massage movements. Because the latissimus dorsi and other lower back muscles extend into the upper back, some of your lower back work will reach the upper back. To avoid injuring the spine and the kidneys, do not do compressions on the lower back.

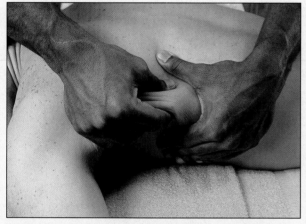

PICK-UP (to latissimus) This Swedish stroke is so beneficial to the muscle that it is often included in a sports massage. Start at your partner's waist and work to underneath his arms.

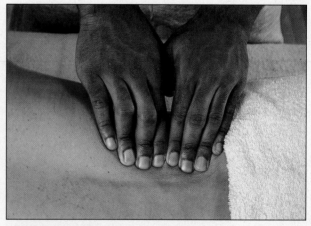

LOCAL CROSS-FIBER (to erectors) Because these narrow muscles are so long, use the fingers of both hands. Work next to the spine from the tailbone to the base of the neck.

BROAD CROSS-FIBER (to latissimus) Place your nonworking hand on your partner's back for stability *(opposite)*. Start the cross-fiber stroke next to his spine, just below the waist. Stroke outward to his side. Move in thumb-length increments until you reach his shoulder blades.

Gluteals

Any sport that requires leg strength, particularly short, fast bursts of running, places extra demands on the gluteals, the broad muscles of the buttocks. The gluteals are one of the largest and strongest muscle groups in the body and have good circulation. As a result, they are less prone to injury than most muscles. But exercise can cause a build-up of lactic acid, which can make the gluteals sore. In addition, they can be affected by tension or injury in the lower back or hamstrings (located in the posterior thigh), which can cause trigger points to develop in the buttocks.

Because of their size and the lack of bone around them, you will be able to work the gluteals thoroughly with the longer and deeper strokes of sports massage. Begin your massage with compressions.

Place a towel over the buttocks you are not massaging; it can extend to cover some of the muscle you are working on as well. When you switch sides, slide the towel over the buttocks you have just finished working on.

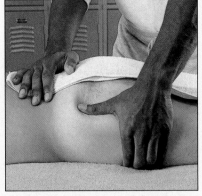

BROAD CROSS-FIBER Start at the bottom of the gluteals. Push deeply into the muscle as you stroke across; work upward.

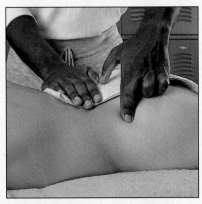

LOCAL CROSS-FIBER (finger-on-finger) Stroke next to the hipbone. Move back and forth, following the line of the bone.

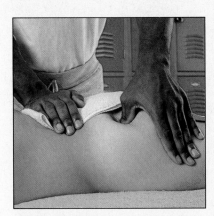

TRIGGER POINTS Search for triggers in the gluteal area. Hold for up to 60 seconds.

DEEP STROKING (thumb-on-thumb) Starting at the hipbone, stroke diagonally down the gluteals *(opposite)*. Progress along the muscle at one-inch intervals.

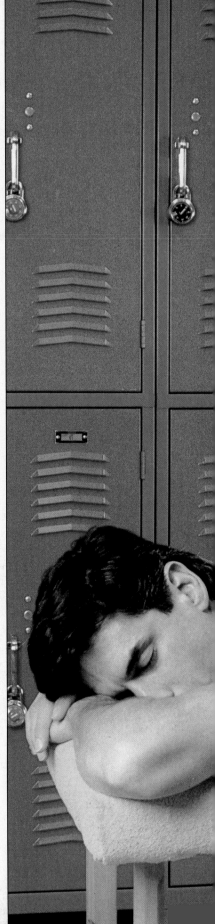

110

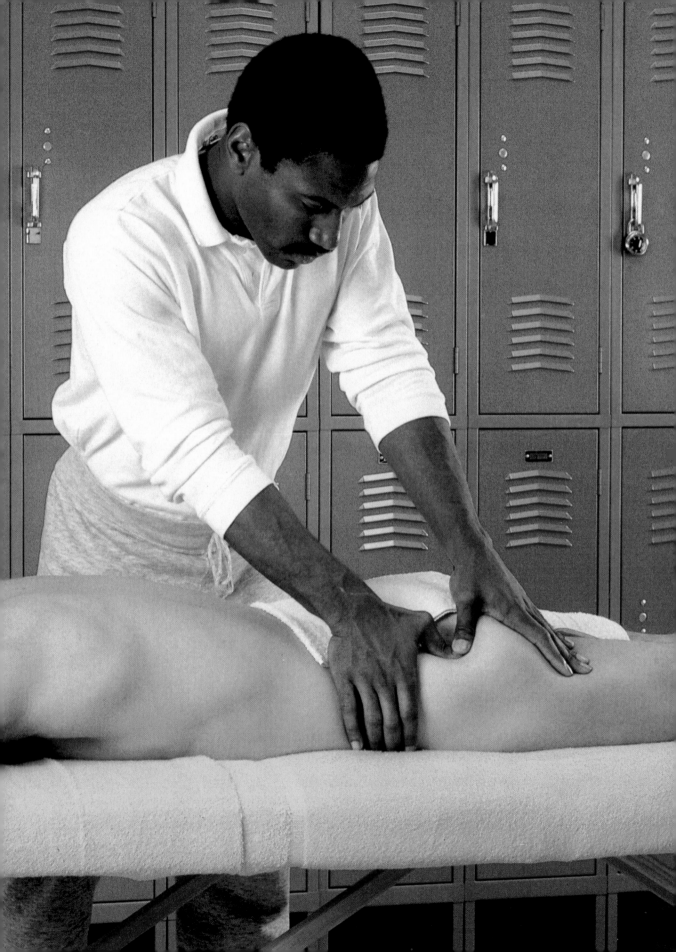

Posterior Thigh

The hamstrings — the major muscles of the posterior thigh — are one of the longest muscle groups in the body, extending from the lower pelvis to the knee. They are one of the sites most vulnerable to athletic injury. A pulled hamstring, a common runners' complaint, results from overexertion and overstretching, which inhibit the muscle's ability to relax. Massage will relax the muscle and remove built-up lactic acid. When combined with stretching, these techniques will help keep the muscle flexible.

Because these muscles are usually strong and large, massaging them can be strenuous. Intersperse your deeper work with jostling, which will relax both your partner's hamstrings and your hands.

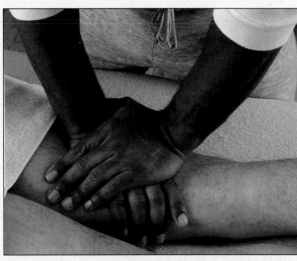

COMPRESSIONS (hand-on-hand) Start several inches below the buttocks. Avoid the back of the knee and its tendons.

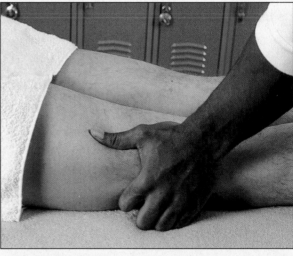

BROAD CROSS-FIBER Work from the knees to the gluteals, first stroking outward, then inward with your other hand.

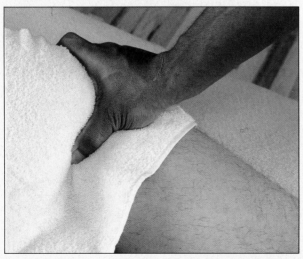

TRIGGER POINTS Search for triggers where the hamstrings meet the gluteals. Clamp your hand around the leg for extra pressure.

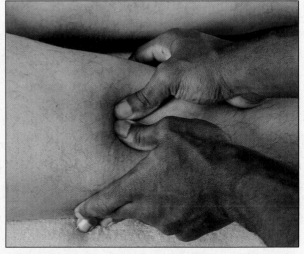

DEEP STROKING (two-thumb) Work from the knees to the gluteals, avoiding the tendons. Repeat at thumb-wide intervals.

JOSTLING Place your hands on either side of the thigh and lift the muscle from the bone as you gently shake it up and down its length *(opposite)*.

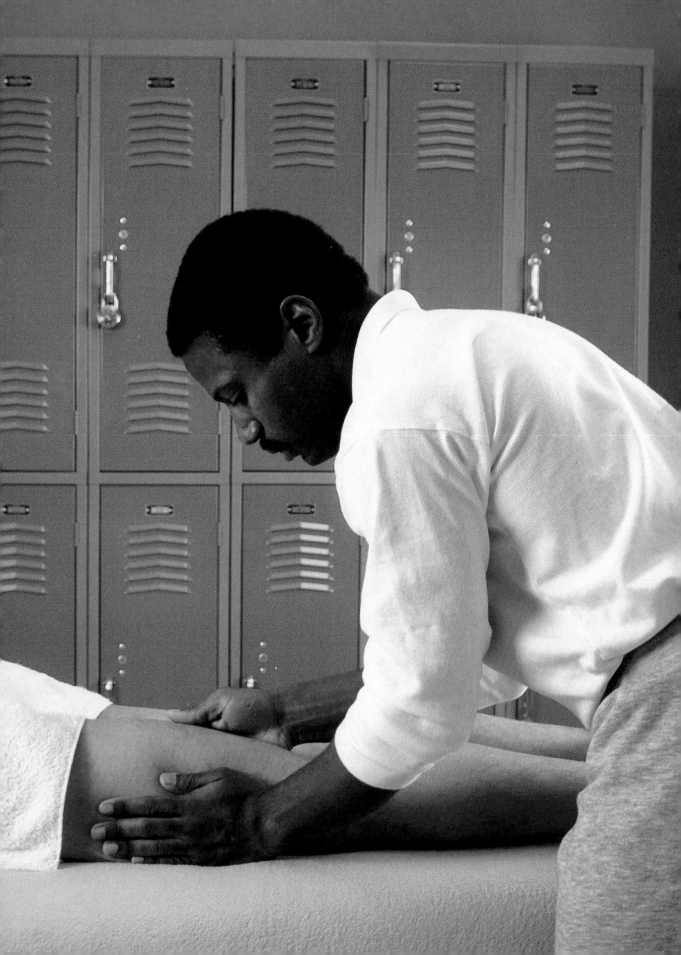

Calf

Each time you take a step, you use muscles and tendons in the calf. The gastrocnemius, the major calf muscle, attaches to the Achilles tendon about two thirds of the way down the calf. This tendon — the largest in the body — is one of the most frequently injured sites in the body. The strain that everyday use imposes on the Achilles tendon can easily beome excessive when you participate in demanding sports.

Certain exercises that work the leg can tighten the gastrocnemius, which in turn pulls on the Achilles tendon. In addition, the gastrocnemius itself is prone to small tears and adhesions from constant use.

Broad cross-fiber stroking to the calf muscles will keep muscle fibers separated, improving muscle flexibility and easing the strain on the Achilles tendon. Use only local cross-fiber stroking when massaging the Achilles tendon; heavy longitudinal strokes like the deep stroke can cause tendinitis, a painful inflammation of the tendons.

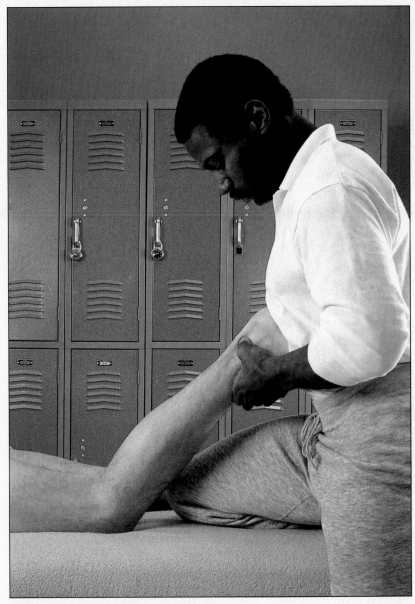

LOCAL CROSS-FIBER (to Achilles tendon)
Bend your partner's foot to stretch his Achilles tendon and press his sole to your stomach. Cup your hands around his ankle. Work across the tendon with your thumbs, moving down its entire length.

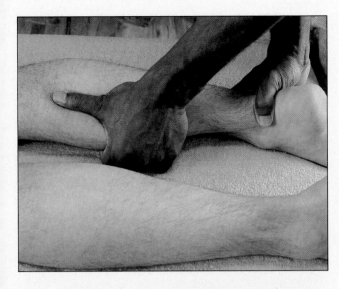

BROAD CROSS-FIBER Hold your partner's right ankle with your right hand and use your left hand to stroke from the center of the calf to the inside. Work up the length of the muscle; then switch hands and stroke from the center to the outside.

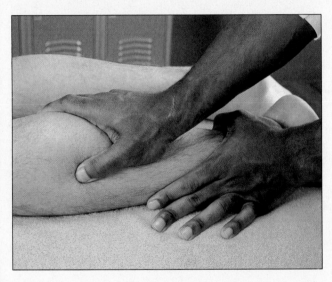

DEEP STROKING Hold your partner's left ankle with your left hand for stability. Grasp his calf with your right hand and stroke deeply up the muscle with your thumb. Start on the outside of the muscle, and work around to the inside.

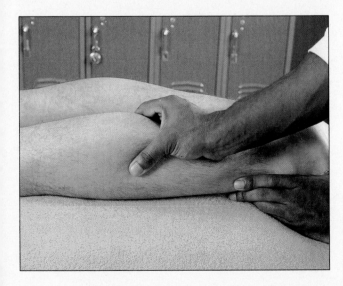

JOSTLING Hold your partner's foot for stability. Grasp the calf muscle between the thumb and fingers of your other hand, and shake back and forth rhythmically. Move up and down the muscle several times, but avoid the Achilles tendon.

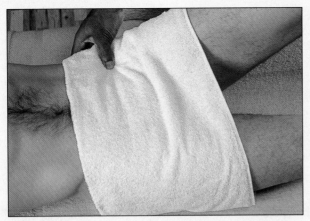

LOCAL CROSS-FIBER (one-thumb) Bend your partner's leg up to help you locate the tendon between the hip and thigh. Grasp the outside of your partner's hip, and work across the tendon.

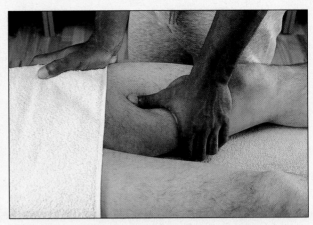

BROAD CROSS-FIBER (to hamstrings) Place your left hand above your partner's knee so that your thumb points toward his hip. Roll inward. Work to the hip, then roll out with your right hand.

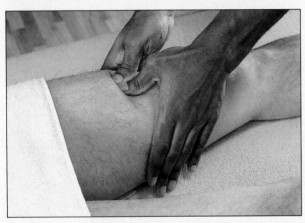

DEEP STROKING (joined-thumb) Place your hands on either side of your partner's thigh, avoiding the tendons. Stroke up to the hip; return and work around the muscle at one-inch intervals.

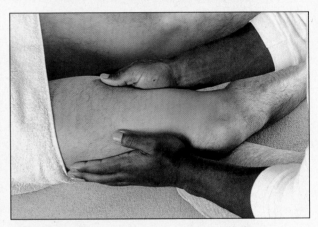

JOSTLING Bend your partner's knee slightly and place your hands on either side of his thigh. Work vigorously to involve all the thigh muscles as you jostle up and down the thigh.

Anterior Thigh

The largest muscle in the body, the quadriceps is a four-part muscle that runs down the front of the thigh from the hip to the knee. Essential to all forward movement, the quadriceps is particularly important in activities like sprinting, racquet sports and soccer, which require sudden bursts of speed. The anterior thigh also contains the adductors, or groin muscles, which lie on the inside of the thigh between the hamstrings and quadriceps.

Overexercised, tight quadriceps and adductors pull on the adjacent hip and knee joints. Massaging these muscles will lengthen them, helping them function more effectively as well as reducing strain on the joints. Massaging the tendons and ligaments of the joints themselves will also improve joint flexibility.

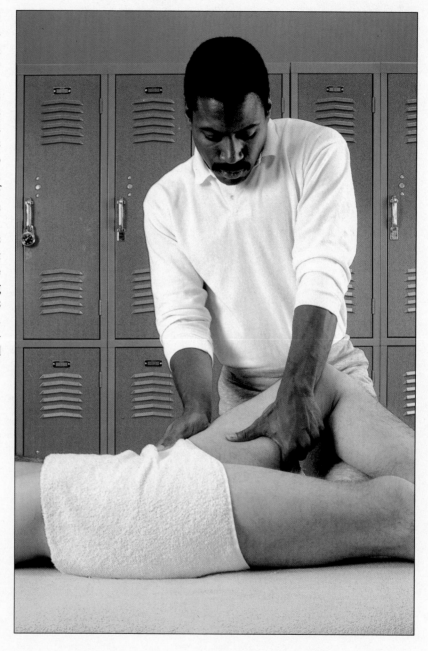

BROAD CROSS-FIBER (to adductors) Bend your partner's leg outward and rest it on your bent knee. Place your hand on the inside of his thigh, with your thumb pointing to the hip, and roll downward. Start above the knee and work up the muscle toward the groin.

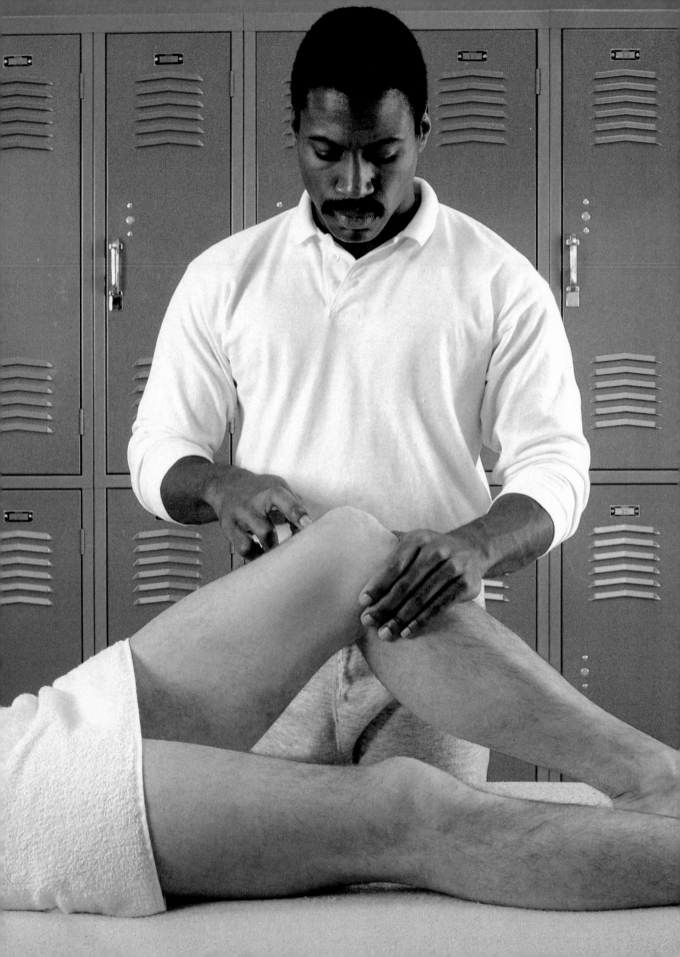

Knee and Shin

The muscles of both the upper and lower leg meet at the knee, an injury-prone joint. You can lessen the likelihood of knee injury by massaging the leg muscles to keep them long and supple, and performing local cross-fiber to the tendons and ligaments adjoining the knee. Massage can also help prevent shin splints, which occur when the shin muscles pull away from the tibia, or shinbone, due to fatigued and irritated muscles and tendons (usually a result of over-training). It is very important, though, to massage toward the shinbone, not away from it.

LOCAL CROSS-FIBER (to knee) Bend your partner's left leg up *(opposite)*. Use two fingers to work across the tendon above the knee. Switch hands and work across the ligament just below the knee.

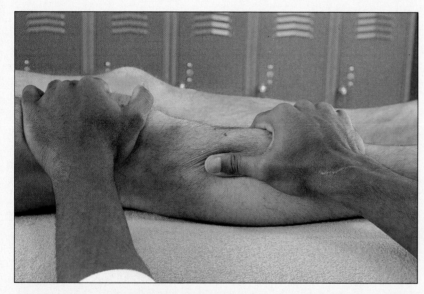

BROAD CROSS-FIBER (to calf) Grasp your partner's calf just above the ankle so that your thumb is on the outside. Roll your thumb up toward the bone; gradually work toward the knee. (Never pull the shin muscle away from the bone.)

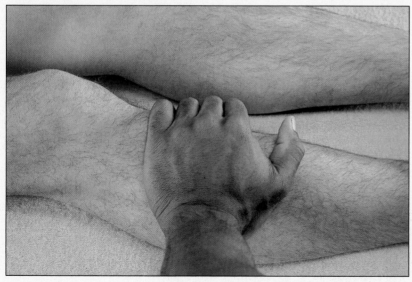

COMPRESSIONS (one-hand) Grasp your partner's calf just above the ankle. Squeeze up and down with your palm on the outer portion of the shin. Do not exert pressure on the shinbone itself. Work up to below the knee and back down.

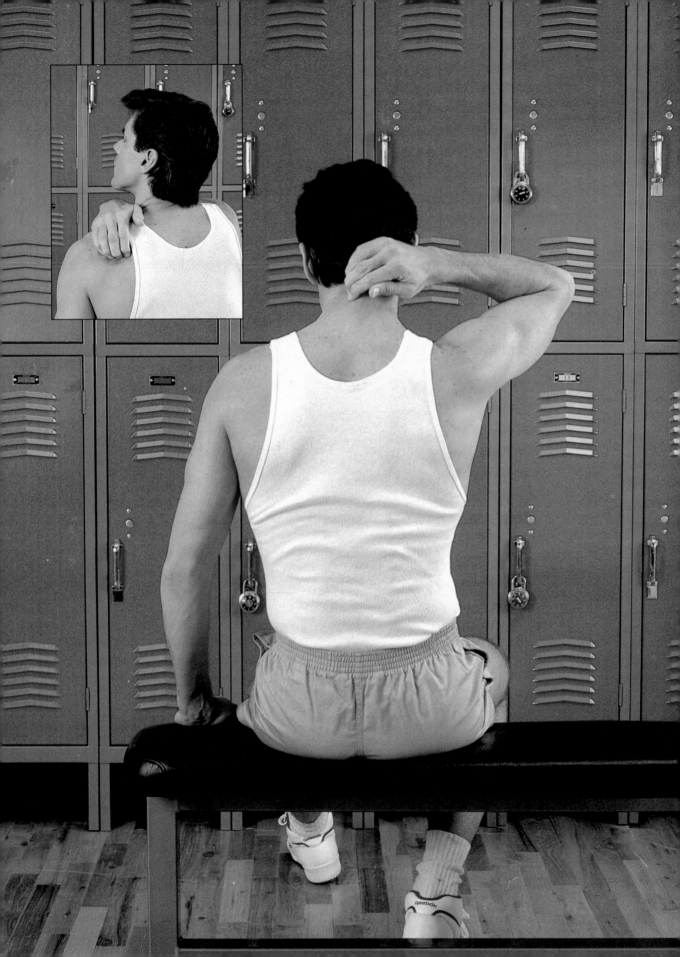

Self-Massage/Upper Body

Self-massage is particularly appropriate in sports massage, since it can provide immediate relief from sudden aches and can alleviate postworkout soreness when a massage partner is unavailable.

You should use self-massage as an adjunct to, not as a substitute for, massage by a partner. Effective sports massage works deeply into the muscles; achieving the same depth when massaging yourself is almost impossible. Because you cannot put your body's strength into the strokes, you do not have the leverage needed for some techniques, such as compressions and broad cross-fiber and deep stroking — particularly when self-massaging the upper body. Instead, concentrate on local cross-fiber strokes, incorporating other techniques as much as possible.

You can sit on the floor or on a bench to perform these techniques.

LOCAL CROSS-FIBER (neck and upper back) Place the fingers of your right hand on the far side of your neck bone *(opposite)*. Rotate them. Then bring your arm over your shoulder *(inset)* and rotate your fingers above your shoulder blade. Repeat with your left hand.

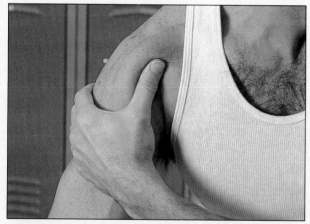

BROAD CROSS-FIBER (deltoids) Grasp your right arm below the shoulder with your left hand. Roll outward with your thumb, working upward.

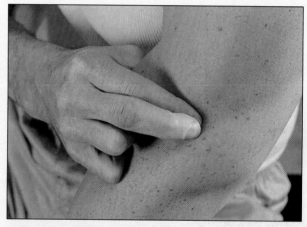

LOCAL CROSS-FIBER (finger-on-finger to elbow) With your elbow slightly bent, locate the tendons just above it and move your fingers back and forth across them.

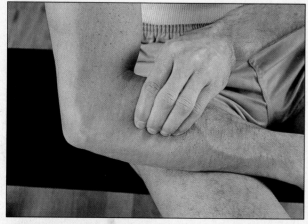

LOCAL CROSS-FIBER (four fingers to forearm) Bend your arm in your lap for support. Rotate your fingers to work across the tendons and muscles of your forearm.

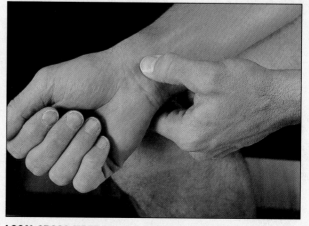

LOCAL CROSS-FIBER (to wrist) Bend your wrist back and use your thumb to work across the flexor tendon inside the wrist; then bend your wrist forward and massage the tendon on the outside.

Self-Massage/ Lower Body

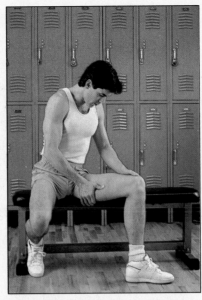

Generally, self-massage is most effective on the lower body. The muscles of the lower body are easier to reach than those of the upper body, and you can use both arms for leverage, which allows you to work into the muscles more deeply. Also, because the muscles of the lower body are both longer and broader, you can use more broad cross-fiber stroking.

You will have difficulty massaging hard-to-reach areas like the back of your thighs, your gluteals or your back. Concentrate instead on the quadriceps and adductors on the front and inside of your thighs, and the muscles and tendons of your knees and lower legs.

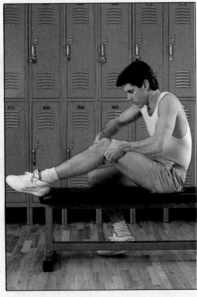

LOCAL CROSS-FIBER (to hip joint) Sit with your left hip slightly extended. Rotate the fingers of your left hand around the joint.

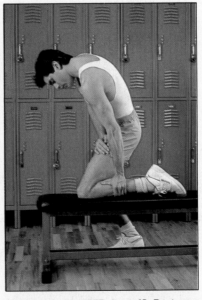

BROAD CROSS-FIBER (to adductors) Extend your left leg. Grasp the inside of your thigh, and roll out with your thumb.

LOCAL CROSS-FIBER (to knee) Bend your knee slightly and grip above and below the joint. Move your thumbs back and forth.

BROAD CROSS-FIBER (to calf) Rest your bent knee on a surface so that your calf is behind you. Grasp the calf and roll out.

LOCAL CROSS-FIBER (to instep) Bend your knee. The ligaments here run crosswise, so work up and down with your thumb *(opposite)*. Also, bend your ankle to point your toes upward, and work your thumb back and forth along the Achilles tendon.

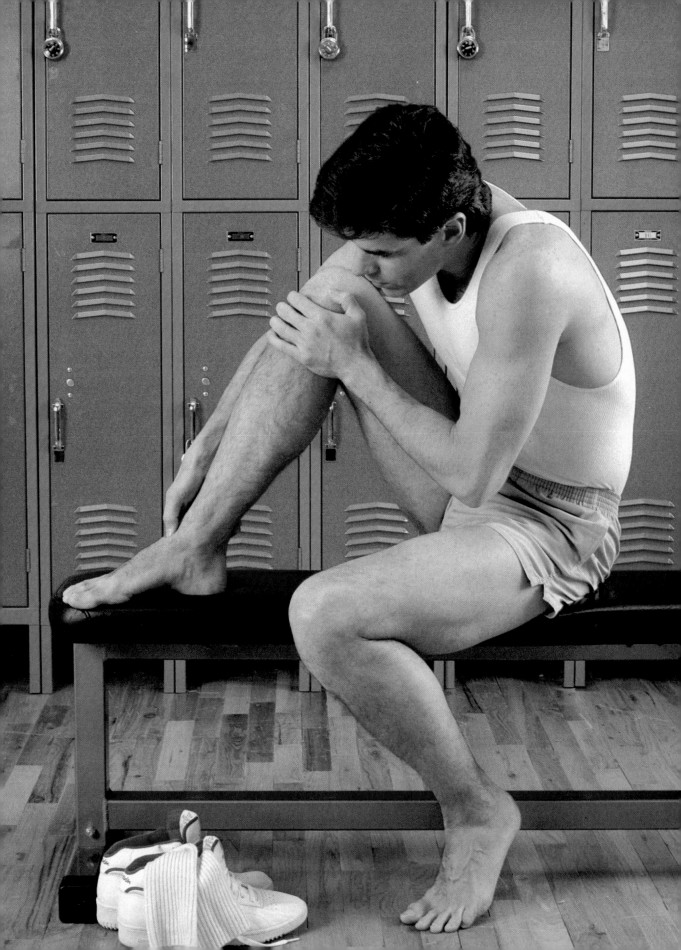

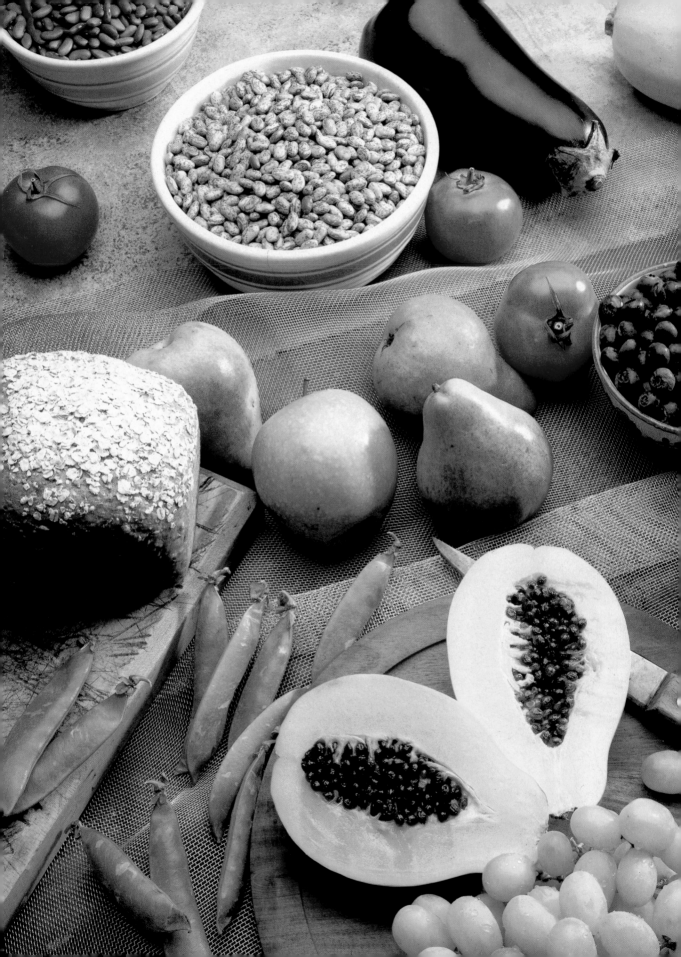

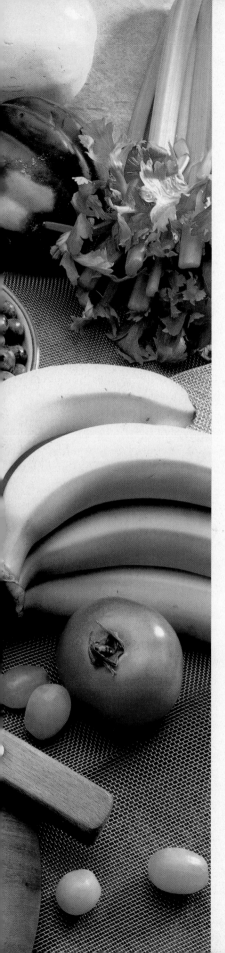

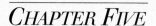
Fiber

More than just bran, with benefits for your digestion, weight control and cholesterol level

F iber, the indigestible but edible part of a plant, is vital to good health and important to good nutrition. Although it is not an essential nutrient, as are protein, carbohydrate and fat, fiber aids in the regulation of basic bodily functions, can help lower cholesterol levels, and may prevent certain intestinal diseases, including colon cancer. It can even contribute to weight control.

Just as a good massage helps to ease muscular tension and to rid muscles of lactic acid, so some types of fiber ease the passage of waste products through your digestive system. For example, by promoting more efficient elimination, the fiber in the bran in whole grains, when consumed with enough fluid, helps regulate bowel function and can prevent or cure constipation.

Contrary to popular belief, bran is not the only source of fiber. In fact, if you limit your high-fiber foods to dishes containing bran or whole-grain breads, you will short-change yourself nutritionally. The term "fiber" actually refers to widely different chemical substances

125

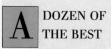

A DOZEN OF THE BEST

The following foods are all high in fiber.

LEGUMES
Lentils
Peas

GRAINS
Bran cereal
Wheat and oat bran

VEGETABLES
Broccoli
Carrots
Potatoes (with skins)
Squash
Turnips

FRUITS
Apples
Berries
Prunes

with different health benefits. And although fiber is frequently called bulk or roughage, some types, such as those found in strawberries and tomatoes, are soft and moist. The various fibers can be divided into two major groups — water-insoluble and water-soluble. Most plant foods contain fibers from both groups, but generally a food is higher in one type of fiber than the other.

Water-insoluble fiber includes cellulose and hemicellulose, both found in the cell walls of plants, and lignin, which makes up the woody part of plants. Wheat bran is an insoluble fiber, consisting of the outer protective layer of a grain of wheat. Insoluble fiber can also be found on the outside of most seeds, nuts, dried beans and peas, and in many vegetables and fruits; however, it is frequently removed when food is processed by milling, peeling, boiling or extracting.

The laxative power of insoluble fiber results from its spongelike action in the gastrointestinal tract. It absorbs many times its weight in water, forming stools that are soft and bulky, and thus capable of being swept quickly through the intestines. Insoluble fiber also reduces pressure on the intestinal walls, which can help prevent diverticulosis, the formation of tiny pouches in the intestine. When these pouches become inflamed, the result is diverticulitis, a painful condition that affects about one person in three over age 60.

Insoluble fiber may reduce the presence of bacteria in the gut that interact with fat and bile acids to produce carcinogens. Because such fiber speeds the movement of food through the colon, it has the ability to flush a variety of potential carcinogens from the body. Some scientists believe that this may partly explain why colon cancer is rare among populations with a diet low in fat and high in fiber. So although the evidence is inconclusive, insoluble fiber may protect you against colon cancer, the second most common cancer in adults.

Water-soluble fiber occurs in pectin, which is found mainly in fruits, particularly apples and berries; in gums, found primarily in oat bran and soybeans, chickpeas and other legumes; and in mucilages, common in many seeds. Pectin and gums delay movement of food from the stomach to the small intestine and control the rate of conversion of carbohydrates to blood sugar. These qualities may help stabilize blood-sugar levels, which is of value in treating diabetes. Soluble fibers may also offer protection against heart disease: Studies have shown that oats and legumes can significantly decrease the level of artery-clogging cholesterol in the blood.

The daily dietary fiber intake in the United States averages about five to 10 grams per person, but the National Cancer Institute and the American Dietetic Association recommend an intake of 25 to 35 grams. This amount is easy to consume if you eat a variety of foods: A cup of bran cereal can have from five to 25 grams of dietary fiber; half a cup of cooked lentils and a large raw carrot have four grams each; a small unpeeled apple has three grams. (Although there is no one method for measuring fiber, the measurement presently accepted by nutritionists is dietary fiber, which represents all indigestible carbohy-

The Basic Guidelines

For a moderately active adult, the National Institutes of Health recommends a diet that is low in fat, high in carbohydrates and moderate in protein. The institutes' guidelines suggest that no more than 30 percent of your calories come from fat, that 55 to 60 percent come from carbohydrates and that no more than 15 percent come from protein. A gram of fat equals nine calories, while a gram of protein or carbohydrate equals four calories; therefore, if you eat 2,100 calories a day, you should consume approximately 60 grams of fat, 315 grams of carbohydrate and no more than 75 grams of protein daily. If you follow a lowfat/high-carbohydrate diet, your chance of developing heart disease, cancer and other life-threatening diseases may be considerably reduced.

◆ The nutrition charts that accompany each of the lowfat/high-carbohydrate recipes in this book include the number of calories per serving, the number of grams of fat, carbohydrate and protein in a serving, and the percentage of calories derived from each of these nutrients. In addition, the charts provide the amount of calcium, iron and sodium per serving.

◆ Calcium deficiency may be associated with periodontal disease — which attacks the mouth's bones and tissues, including the gums — in both men and women, and with osteoporosis, or bone shrinking and weakening, in the elderly. The deficiency may also contribute to high blood pressure. The recommended daily allowance for calcium is 800 milligrams a day for men and women. Pregnant and lactating women are advised to consume 1,200 milligrams daily; a National Institutes of Health consensus panel recommends that postmenopausal women consume 1,200 to 1,500 milligrams of calcium daily.

◆ Although one way you can reduce your fat intake is to cut your consumption of red meat, you should make sure that you get your necessary iron from other sources. The Food and Nutrition Board of the National Academy of Sciences suggests a minimum of 10 milligrams of iron per day for men and 18 milligrams for women between the ages of 11 and 50.

◆ High sodium intake is associated with high blood pressure. Most adults should restrict sodium intake to between 2,000 and 2,500 milligrams a day, according to the National Academy of Sciences. One way to keep sodium consumption in check is not to add table salt to food.

drates in food.) Because fiber fills you up without adding calories and because fibrous foods take longer to chew, a high-fiber regimen may aid in weight control. Moreover, because it expands quickly in the stomach and small intestine, soluble fiber makes you feel full longer.

If your diet is low in fiber, increase your intake gradually; consuming too much fiber too soon can cause intestinal gas or diarrhea and irritate the intestinal lining. Also, excessive fiber intake can interfere with the absorption of calcium, iron, magnesium and other minerals. But if your diet is well balanced, this should not be a problem.

As a rule, the less processed food you consume, the higher your fiber intake. Raw fruits and vegetables contain more useful fiber than those that have been canned or otherwise processed. Unpeeled produce is higher in fiber than peeled fruits and vegetables. The recipes that follow provide fiber in its most nutritious forms in a variety of dishes, including beverages and desserts.

Breakfast

PRUNE BRAN MUFFINS

Oat bran is a good choice for those who want to increase their dietary fiber intake gradually, since it is relatively easy on the digestive system.

Vegetable cooking spray
2 1/2 cups oat bran
1 tablespoon baking powder
1/4 teaspoon salt
2/3 cup skim milk

2 eggs, beaten
1/3 cup honey
2 tablespoons safflower oil
10 pitted prunes, chopped

Preheat the oven to 425° F. Spray 12 muffin tin cups with cooking spray, or line them with paper liners. In a large bowl combine the bran, baking powder and salt. Add the milk, eggs, honey and oil, and stir until just combined; do not overmix the batter. Stir in the prunes. Divide the batter among the muffin tin cups and bake 20 to 25 minutes, or until a toothpick inserted in a muffin comes out clean.   Makes 12 muffins

CALORIES per muffin	163
58% Carbohydrate	24 g
13% Protein	6 g
29% Fat	5 g
CALCIUM	92 mg
IRON	1 mg
SODIUM	171 mg

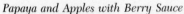

Papaya and Apples with Berry Sauce

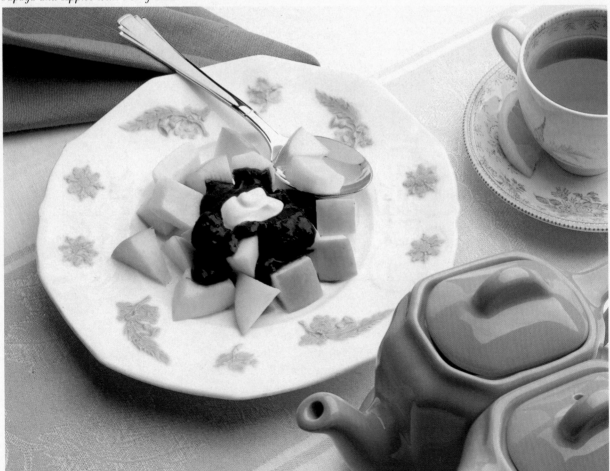

CRANBERRY-RAISIN BREAD

A study of overweight college men on a restricted-calorie diet showed that those who ate a high-fiber bread like this one daily lost more weight than those who consumed the same amount of ordinary white bread.

CALORIES per slice	164
78% Carbohydrate	32 g
7% Protein	3 g
15% Fat	3 g
CALCIUM	38 mg
IRON	1 mg
SODIUM	208 mg

Vegetable cooking spray
2 cups unbleached all-purpose
 flour
1/2 cup sugar
1 1/2 teaspoons baking powder
1/2 teaspoon baking soda
1/2 teaspoon salt

2 tablespoons butter or margarine
3/4 cup white grape juice
1 egg, beaten
1 cup coarsely chopped cranberries
1/2 cup raisins
1 tablespoon grated lemon peel

Preheat the oven to 350° F. Spray a 9 x 5-inch loaf pan with cooking spray and dust it lightly with flour. In a large bowl combine the remaining flour, the sugar, baking powder, baking soda and salt. Using a pastry blender or two knives, cut in the butter until the mixture resembles coarse meal. Stir in the grape juice and egg, then fold in the cranberries, raisins and lemon peel. Pour the batter into the prepared pan and bake it for about 1 hour, or until a toothpick inserted into the loaf comes out clean. Cut the loaf into 12 slices.

Makes 12 servings

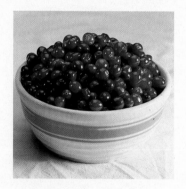

Note: The cranberries can be chopped in a food processor or with a curved chopper in a wooden bowl. The bread can be made with purple grape juice, but it will have a slight bluish cast.

PAPAYA AND APPLES WITH BERRY SAUCE

The peel of the apple contributes a considerable amount of insoluble fiber to this refreshing low-calorie breakfast dish. Cook with and eat unpeeled apples whenever possible.

1 papaya
1 Granny Smith apple
2 teaspoons lemon juice
1 cup fresh or unsweetened
 frozen blackberries
 or raspberries

2 teaspoons Cointreau (optional)
1 teaspoon honey
2 tablespoons nonbutterfat sour
 dressing

CALORIES per serving	89
82% Carbohydrate	20 g
4% Protein	1 g
14% Fat	2 g
CALCIUM	35 mg
IRON	.3 mg
SODIUM	6 mg

Peel the papaya, seed it and cut it into 1/2-inch cubes. Core but do not peel the apple and cut it into 1/2-inch cubes. Place the apple cubes in a large bowl and toss them with the lemon juice; set aside. Combine the berries, Cointreau, if using, and honey in a blender, and process until just combined. Add the papaya cubes to the apple cubes and toss; divide the mixture among 4 plates. Spoon the berry sauce over the fruit and top each serving with 1 1/2 teaspoons of sour dressing.

Makes 4 servings

Lunch

. . . .

SPINACH AND TOFU SALAD

Spinach and bell peppers supply the fiber in this Japanese-inspired side dish. This salad also provides high-quality, lowfat protein and more than 25 percent of a woman's daily iron requirement.

CALORIES per serving	59
42% Carbohydrate	7g
32% Protein	6 g
26% Fat	2 g
CALCIUM	158 mg
IRON	5 mg
SODIUM	361 mg

20 ounces spinach, with stems
1 ounce firm tofu, finely chopped
  (6 tablespoons)
1 red bell pepper, thinly sliced
2 large scallions, finely chopped

1 tablespoon plus 1 teaspoon
  tamari
1 teaspoon Oriental sesame oil
1/2 teaspoon black pepper

Trim the roots from the spinach, if necessary, but leave the stems intact. Wash the spinach thoroughly but do not dry it. Place the spinach in a large saucepan over medium heat, cover and cook, stirring occasionally to ensure even cooking, 3 to 5 minutes, or until the spinach is just wilted. Drain the spinach, rinse it under cold water and squeeze out any excess moisture with your hands; pat dry with paper towels. Place the spinach in a large serving bowl and toss it with a fork to separate it. Add the remaining ingredients and toss to combine. Divide the salad among 4 plates.   Makes 4 servings

Note: Tamari is a mellow, somewhat sweet unrefined soy sauce. Look for it in Oriental food shops, health-food stores and many supermarkets.

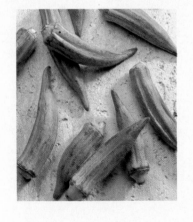

VEGETABLE GUMBO

Tomatoes, okra and bell peppers, traditional ingredients of the Creole stew called gumbo, provide most of the fiber here. Vegetables like cucumbers and lettuce, which are mostly water, are low in fiber by comparison.

2 tablespoons unbleached
  all-purpose flour
1 tablespoon vegetable oil
3 cups canned plum tomatoes
1 cup coarsely chopped onion
1 cup coarsely chopped green bell
  pepper
1 cup chopped celery
1/2 teaspoon dried thyme

1 bay leaf
1/4 teaspoon hot pepper sauce, or
  to taste
2 tablespoons chopped fresh
  parsley
1/4 teaspoon salt
1/4 teaspoon black pepper
10 ounces whole okra, trimmed

CALORIES per serving	120
59% Carbohydrate	19 g
12% Protein	4 g
29% Fat	4 g
CALCIUM	106 mg
IRON	3 mg
SODIUM	468 mg

Stir the flour and oil together in a medium-size saucepan over medium heat for about 2 minutes, or until the flour is browned. Add the tomatoes and their liquid, the onion, bell pepper, celery, thyme, bay leaf, hot pepper sauce, parsley, salt and pepper. Reduce the heat to low and simmer, uncovered, 20 minutes. Add the okra and cook another 10 minutes. Remove and discard the bay leaf, then ladle the gumbo into 4 bowls and serve.   Makes 4 servings

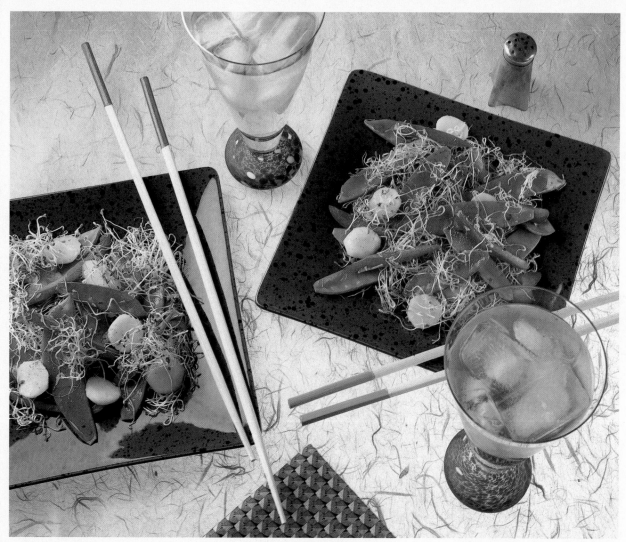

Oriental Salad

ORIENTAL SALAD

*Blanching vegetables like snow peas preserves more of their fiber than
prolonged boiling, which breaks down the fiber. Quick cooking also keeps
their texture crisp and their color bright.*

3/4 pound snow peas, blanched

1/4 pound alfalfa sprouts

1 cup thinly sliced red bell pepper

One 3 1/2-ounce can water
   chestnuts, drained and sliced

1/3 cup Japanese rice-wine vinegar

2 teaspoons Oriental sesame oil

1/4 teaspoon black pepper

Pinch of salt

CALORIES per serving	86
56% Carbohydrate	13 g
17% Protein	4 g
27% Fat	3 g
CALCIUM	49 mg
IRON	3 mg
SODIUM	44 mg

In a large bowl toss together the snow peas, sprouts, bell pepper and water
chestnuts. Add the vinegar, oil, pepper and salt, and toss to combine.

Makes 4 servings

SPICY VEGETABLE SAUTE

Using fresh tomatoes and potatoes with their skins adds fiber to this dish.

CALORIES per serving	149
68% Carbohydrate	27 g
10% Protein	4 g
22% Fat	4 g
CALCIUM	44 mg
IRON	3 mg
SODIUM	49 mg

2 medium-size baking potatoes
1 tablespoon vegetable oil
5 fresh plum tomatoes
10 ounces green beans, cut into
  1-inch pieces (2 cups)

1 small red onion, sliced
2 teaspoons turmeric
1/2 teaspoon red pepper flakes
Pinch of salt
Pinch of black pepper

Preheat the oven to 400° F. Scrub but do not peel the potatoes and cut them into 1/4-inch dice. Place the potatoes on a foil-lined baking sheet, toss them with 1 teaspoon of oil and bake, turning occasionally with a spatula, 15 to 20 minutes, or until golden. Meanwhile, wash and coarsely dice the tomatoes.

    In a medium-size skillet over medium heat, sauté the tomatoes, beans and onion in the remaining oil about 5 minutes, or just until tender. Add the potatoes and seasonings and stir gently to combine.   Makes 4 servings

TOSSED SALAD WITH CITRUS-MUSTARD DRESSING

The beans in this salad are a good source of water-soluble gums, a type of fiber that lowers blood cholesterol.

CALORIES per serving	90
65% Carbohydrate	15 g
19% Protein	4 g
16% Fat	2 g
CALCIUM	33 mg
IRON	2 mg
SODIUM	187 mg

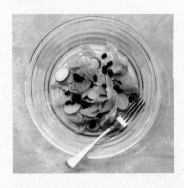

1/3 cup grapefruit juice, preferably
  freshly squeezed
1 teaspoon sunflower oil
1 teaspoon Dijon-style mustard
1/4 teaspoon salt
1/4 teaspoon pepper

10 radishes, thinly sliced
1 carrot, thinly sliced
3 1/2 ounces butter lettuce, torn
  into bite-size pieces
1/3 cup cooked black beans

For the dressing, in a small bowl stir together the grapefruit juice, oil, mustard, salt and pepper; set aside. Combine the remaining ingredients in a large bowl. Pour the dressing over the salad and toss to combine.   Makes 4 servings

BLACK BEAN AND ORANGE SOUP

Carrots are rich in both soluble and insoluble fiber.

CALORIES per serving	186
78% Carbohydrate	39 g
18% Protein	9 g
4% Fat	1 g
CALCIUM	88 mg
IRON	3 mg
SODIUM	23 mg

1 1/2 cups orange juice, preferably
  freshly squeezed
1 1/4 cups cooked black beans
  (5/8 cup dried)

2 carrots, cut into 3-inch pieces
1 cup finely chopped onion
1 teaspoon ground coriander
4 orange slices, for garnish

Place the juice, beans, carrots, onion and coriander in a medium-size nonreactive saucepan. Bring to a boil, reduce the heat to low and simmer, covered, 20 minutes. Set the soup aside to cool briefly, then process it in a food processor or blender just until puréed. Reheat the soup over low heat, then ladle it into 4 bowls and garnish with orange slices.   Makes 4 servings

Dinner

AFRICAN CURRY WITH BROWN RICE

Studies indicate that the typical African diet, which includes many high-fiber vegetable dishes similar to this one, is probably an important factor in the low incidence of colon cancer on that continent.

1 cup brown rice	1/2 cup sliced onion
One 35-ounce can plum tomatoes	2 tablespoons curry powder
14 ounces unpeeled sweet potatoes, washed and cut into 1/2-inch-thick slices	20 pitted prunes
	1 cup coarsely chopped scallions
	1/2 cup chopped fresh coriander
4 garlic cloves, crushed and peeled	2 tablespoons peanut butter
	1/4 teaspoon salt

CALORIES per serving	515
80% Carbohydrate	109 g
9% Protein	12 g
11% Fat	7 g
CALCIUM	172 mg
IRON	6 mg
SODIUM	600 mg

Bring 2 1/2 cups of water to a boil in a medium-size saucepan. Stir in the rice, cover, reduce the heat to low and cook 45 minutes, or until the rice is tender and the water is completely absorbed. Meanwhile, place the tomatoes and their liquid, the potatoes, garlic, onion and curry powder in a large saucepan. Bring to a boil over medium-high heat, reduce the heat to medium-low and simmer 20 minutes, or until the potatoes are tender. Stir in the remaining ingredients and cook, stirring occasionally, 10 minutes. Divide the rice among 4 plates and top with the curry.   Makes 4 servings

African Curry with Brown Rice

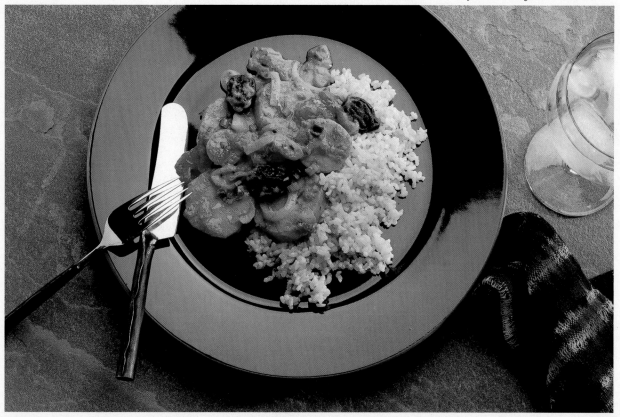

CHILI VEGETABLE SOUP

CALORIES per serving	113
80% Carbohydrate	23 g
15% Protein	5 g
5% Fat	1 g
CALCIUM	62 mg
IRON	2 mg
SODIUM	155 mg

Many rich soups are thickened with cream or a butter-flour mixture, neither of which contains fiber. But puréeing some of the vegetables in this soup produces a satisfying texture without adding fat or calories.

1 pound all-purpose potatoes, peeled and diced (2 1/2 cups)
1 cup frozen corn kernels
1 cup unpeeled, sliced zucchini
3/4 cup coarsely chopped celery
3/4 cup sliced carrot
1/2 cup chopped scallions
1/2 cup coarsely chopped onion
2 garlic cloves, crushed and peeled
2 cups low-sodium chicken stock
1/2 cup skim milk
1 tablespoon mild chili powder
1/4 teaspoon salt
1/4 teaspoon black pepper

Place all of the vegetables, including the onion and garlic, in a large pot. Add 1 cup of water, the stock, milk, chili powder, salt and pepper, and bring to a boil over medium-high heat. Cover the pot, reduce the heat to low and simmer the vegetables 15 to 20 minutes, or until the potatoes are tender. Remove the pot from the heat and let the soup cool for about 20 minutes. Transfer 2 cups of the cooled soup to a food processor or blender and process until puréed. Return the purée to the pot, stir to recombine and reheat the soup briefly over low heat. Ladle the soup into 6 bowls and serve.   Makes 6 servings

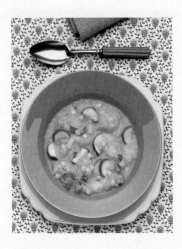

ARTICHOKE SALAD WITH RED CAVIAR DRESSING

Artichokes are high in fiber and low in calories, but they are often served with fatty butter- or mayonnaise-based sauces. This elegant side dish presents the artichokes in a delicious lowfat dressing.

1/4 cup plain lowfat yogurt
1 1/2 cups frozen artichoke hearts, thawed
1/2 pound cherry tomatoes, halved
1/4 cup finely chopped scallions
2 tablespoons nonbutterfat sour dressing
2 teaspoons red caviar, such as salmon or lumpfish
1 teaspoon lemon juice, preferably freshly squeezed
1/4 teaspoon white pepper
4 lemon wedges

CALORIES per serving	66
51% Carbohydrate	9 g
23% Protein	4 g
26% Fat	2 g
CALCIUM	54 mg
IRON	1 mg
SODIUM	111 mg

Line a small strainer with paper towels and set it over a bowl. Pour the yogurt into the strainer and set aside to drain about 10 minutes. Place the artichoke hearts on several layers of paper towels and pat them dry with additional paper towels. (If the artichokes are not thoroughly dried, the salad will be watery.) Place the artichokes in a large bowl and add the tomatoes, scallions, sour dressing, caviar, lemon juice and pepper. Add the drained yogurt and stir gently to combine. Divide the salad among 4 plates, garnish with lemon wedges and serve.   Makes 4 servings

SWEET POTATO AND CARROT PUREE

Sweet potatoes and carrots are two of the richest vegetable sources of fiber, especially when they are unpeeled.

4 medium-size carrots (about
  1 pound total weight)
2 sweet potatoes (about 1 pound
  total weight)

1/2 cup skim milk
2 teaspoons honey
2 teaspoons butter or margarine

CALORIES per serving	206
82% Carbohydrate	43 g
8% Protein	4 g
10% Fat	3 g
CALCIUM	94 mg
IRON	1 mg
SODIUM	93 mg

Wash and trim the carrots but do not peel them; scrub the potatoes but do not peel them. Cut the vegetables into large chunks, then place in a medium-size saucepan with cold water to cover. Bring to a boil over high heat, reduce the heat to low, cover the pan and simmer 20 to 25 minutes, or until the carrots and potatoes are just tender. Transfer the cooked vegetables to a food processor or blender and add the milk, honey and butter. Process the mixture 5 to 10 seconds, or until puréed, turning the machine on and off, and scraping down the sides of the container with a rubber spatula as necessary. Divide the purée among 4 plates and serve.   Makes 4 servings

POACHED CHICKEN WITH GRAPES

Brown rice contains more fiber and vitamin E than processed white rice. Vitamin E is important in the formation of red blood cells.

1 1/4 cups brown rice
1 ounce dried mushrooms, such as
  porcini
2 shallots, thinly sliced
2 tablespoons butter or margarine
4 chicken breast halves with bone
  in, skinned (about 1 1/2 pounds
  total weight)

1 cup coarsely chopped celery
1/2 teaspoon dried thyme
1 bay leaf
Pinch of salt
Pinch of pepper
1/4 cup low-sodium chicken stock
2 cups seedless green grapes
1 teaspoon cornstarch

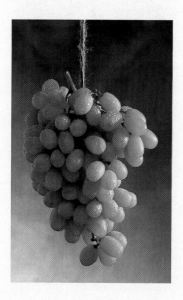

Bring 3 cups of water to a boil in a medium-size saucepan over medium-high heat. Stir in the rice, cover, reduce the heat to low and simmer 45 minutes, or until the rice is tender and the water is completely absorbed. While the rice is cooking, place the mushrooms in a small bowl, pour 1 cup of hot water over them and set aside to soak about 20 minutes.

In a medium-size skillet over medium heat, sauté the shallots in 1 table-spoon of butter for 2 minutes. Add the remaining butter to the skillet, then add the chicken breasts and cook about 2 minutes on each side, or until lightly browned. Strain the mushroom-soaking liquid and add it to the chicken, then add the mushrooms, celery, thyme, bay leaf, salt, pepper and stock. Reduce the heat to low, cover and simmer the chicken 15 to 20 minutes, or until tender. Add 1 1/2 cups of grapes and simmer another 5 minutes.

In a small bowl combine the cornstarch with 1/2 cup cold water and stir well. Stir the cornstarch mixture into the chicken sauce and cook about 2 minutes, or until the sauce is slightly thickened. Divide the rice among 4 plates and place one chicken-breast half on each plate. Spoon the sauce and grapes over the chicken and garnish with the remaining grapes.   Makes 4 servings

CALORIES per serving	491
54% Carbohydrate	66 g
29% Protein	36 g
17% Fat	9 g
CALCIUM	67 mg
IRON	3 mg
SODIUM	224 mg

EGYPTIAN SALAD

CALORIES per serving	112
57% Carbohydrate	17 g
21% Protein	6 g
22% Fat	3 g
CALCIUM	49 mg
IRON	3 mg
SODIUM	61 mg

This recipe is based on an Egyptian dish that is usually made with fava beans and lentils. The kidney beans and green peas used here are, like all legumes, excellent sources of protein and carbohydrate as well as fiber.

4 large Romaine lettuce leaves
1 cup cooked kidney beans (1/2 cup dried)
1 cup frozen green peas, thawed
3/4 cup finely chopped scallions
1/4 cup chopped fresh coriander
2 teaspoons vegetable oil
1 1/2 teaspoons ground cumin
1/2 teaspoon hot pepper sauce

Place a lettuce leaf on each of 4 salad plates. Combine the beans, peas, scallions and coriander in a large bowl and toss gently. Add the oil, cumin and hot pepper sauce and toss again. Spoon the salad onto the lettuce leaves and serve.   Makes 4 servings

SPAGHETTI SQUASH WITH TOMATO SAUCE AND MUSSELS

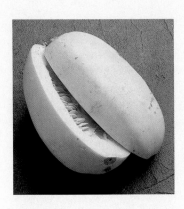

When spaghetti squash is cooked, its flesh separates into spaghetti-like strands to produce a high-fiber, low-calorie substitute for pasta.

1 large spaghetti squash
   (about 2 1/4 pounds)
3 cups canned plum tomatoes,
   with their liquid
1 cup finely chopped onion
2 garlic cloves, crushed and
   peeled
1 bay leaf
1 tablespoon chopped fresh parsley
3/4 teaspoon dried basil
1/4 teaspoon salt
1/4 teaspoon black pepper
8 medium-size mussels,
   cleaned and debearded

CALORIES per serving	76
62% Carbohydrate	13 g
26% Protein	5 g
12% Fat	1 g
CALCIUM	77 mg
IRON	3 mg
SODIUM	502 mg

Preheat the oven to 350° F. Using a large chef's knife or cleaver, halve the squash lengthwise. Remove the seeds and place the squash halves cut side down on a baking sheet. Bake 45 minutes, or until the squash is tender. Meanwhile, for the sauce, in a medium-size nonreactive saucepan combine the tomatoes, onion, garlic, bay leaf, parsley, basil, salt and pepper. Bring the sauce to a boil over medium-high heat, then reduce the heat to low and simmer, uncovered, 35 minutes.

Just before serving, add the mussels to the sauce. Increase the heat to medium, cover the pan and cook the mussels 3 to 5 minutes, or until the shells open. Discard any mussels that do not open. Remove and discard the bay leaf. Remove the squash from the oven and, with 2 forks, pull the strands of flesh from the shell. Mound the squash strands on a serving platter and top with the sauce and mussels.   Makes 4 servings

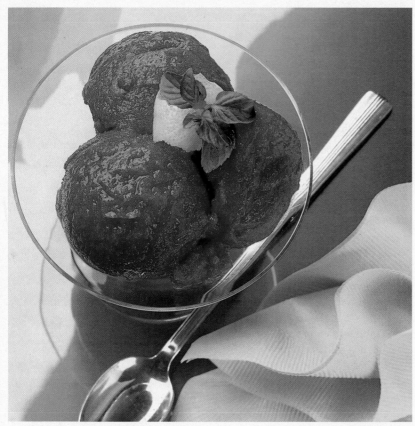

Ruby Sherbet

Desserts

RUBY SHERBET

Pears provide most of the fiber in this colorful dessert.

3 pounds fresh beets
4 1/2 cups pear or apple juice

3 medium-size Bosc pears
1 tablespoon grated lemon peel

Wash, trim, peel and quarter the beets and combine them with the pear juice in a large nonreactive saucepan. Bring to a boil over medium heat, reduce the heat to low and simmer about 15 minutes, or until the beets are tender. Meanwhile, peel, core and halve the pears.

Turn the beets with the cooking liquid into a strainer set over a large bowl. Do not press the beets (reserve them for another use). Return the liquid to the pan, add the pears and lemon peel and simmer over medium heat 5 minutes. Remove the pan from the heat and let the pears cool 20 minutes, then purée the pears and liquid in a food processor or blender. Pour the purée into a shallow pan and freeze 3 hours, or until firm.

Let the sherbet thaw at room temperature for 5 minutes, then scoop it into the food processor or blender and process it about 45 seconds or just until smooth, turning the machine on and off once or twice. Scoop the sherbet into 4 dessert dishes and serve. Makes 4 servings

CALORIES per serving	207
96% Carbohydrate	52 g
1% Protein	1 g
3% Fat	1 g
CALCIUM	36 mg
IRON	1 mg
SODIUM	25 mg

FRUIT LOAF

A study at the University of Kentucky demonstrated that, while beans were as effective as oat bran in lowering blood cholesterol levels, people who ate oat-bran dishes had fewer digestive problems than those who ate beans.

CALORIES per slice	224
72% Carbohydrate	42 g
9% Protein	5 g
19% Fat	5 g
CALCIUM	87 mg
IRON	2 mg
SODIUM	212 mg

Vegetable cooking spray
1 1/2 cups unbleached
   all-purpose flour
1/4 cup apple juice
1 1/2 cups mixed dried fruit,
   coarsely chopped
1 cup oat bran

1 tablespoon baking powder
1/4 teaspoon salt
3 tablespoons butter or margarine,
   softened
1/2 cup honey
2 eggs, beaten
1/2 cup buttermilk

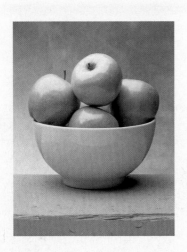

Spray a 9 x 5-inch loaf pan with cooking spray and dust it lightly with flour; set aside. Heat the apple juice in a medium-size nonreactive saucepan over medium heat and stir in the dried fruit. Remove the pan from the heat and set the fruit aside to soak 15 minutes.

In a medium-size bowl stir together the remaining flour, the bran, baking powder and salt. In a large bowl cream together the butter and honey until smooth. Stir in the eggs and buttermilk. Stir in the fruit and apple juice, then add the dry ingredients and stir just until moistened. Turn the batter into the prepared pan and bake 1 hour, or until a toothpick inserted into the loaf comes out clean. When cool, cut the loaf into 12 slices.　　Makes 12 servings

APPLE-APRICOT MOUSSE

Pectin, which is found in many fruits, including apples and apricots, helps give you a satisfying feeling of fullness because it slows the speed at which food leaves your stomach.

2 large Granny Smith apples,
   unpeeled, cored and quartered
10 unsulfured dried apricots

2 tablespoons lemon juice
2 egg whites
1 tablespoon sugar, or less to taste

CALORIES per serving	114
89% Carbohydrate	28 g
8% Protein	3 g
3% Fat	.4 g
CALCIUM	17 mg
IRON	1 mg
SODIUM	28 mg

Combine the apples, apricots, lemon juice and 1/4 cup of water in a medium-size nonreactive saucepan and bring to a boil over medium heat. Reduce the heat to low, cover and simmer 15 to 20 minutes, or until the fruit is tender. Remove the pan from the heat and set the fruit aside to cool for 10 minutes.

Pour the fruit mixture into a food processor or blender and process just until puréed; transfer the purée to a large bowl. In another large bowl, using an electric mixer, beat the egg whites until stiff peaks form, then beat in the sugar. Fold the egg whites gently into the fruit purée. Spoon the mixture into four 4-ounce ramekins or dessert dishes and refrigerate for at least 2 hours, or until set.　　Makes 4 servings

Snacks and Beverages

OPEN-FACED CARROT SALAD SANDWICH

This carrot salad uses banana rather than mayonnaise as a binder because it provides carbohydrates, potassium and fiber — and virtually no fat.

1/2 small banana, peeled

1 medium-size carrot, shredded
  (1 cup)

2 teaspoons lemon juice

1/4 teaspoon grated lemon peel

2 Bibb or butter lettuce leaves

1 slice whole-grain pumpernickel
  bread

2 thin unpeeled apple slices

CALORIES per serving	173
91% Carbohydrate	40 g
5% Protein	4 g
4% Fat	1 g
CALCIUM	73 mg
IRON	2 mg
SODIUM	204 mg

Mash the banana in a small bowl. Add the carrot, lemon juice and lemon peel, and stir to combine. Place the lettuce on the bread, top with the carrot salad and garnish with the apple slices.   Makes 1 serving

Open-Faced Carrot Salad Sandwich

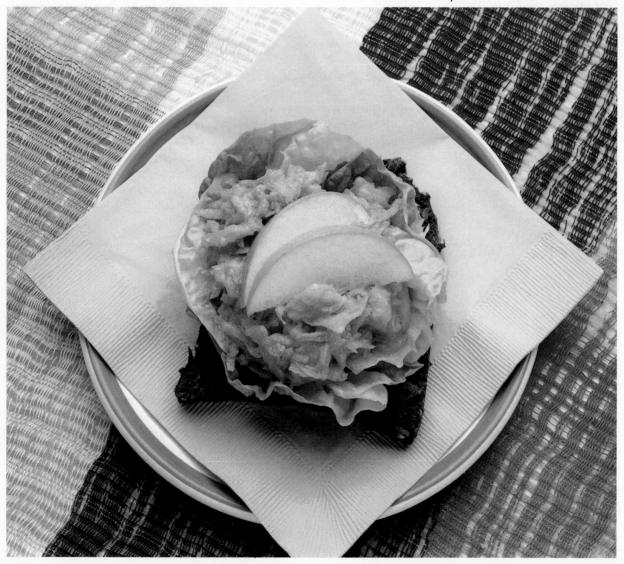

RED LENTIL DIP

Served with an assortment of raw vegetables such as carrots, celery and green beans, this dip makes a filling snack, high in fiber and low in calories.

CALORIES per tablespoon	18
67% Carbohydrate	3 g
29% Protein	1 g
4% Fat	.1 g
CALCIUM	9 mg
IRON	.3 mg
SODIUM	21 mg

1/2 cup red lentils
1/4 cup plain lowfat yogurt
2 tablespoons medium-hot bottled salsa

1 tablespoon chopped fresh chives
Dash of hot pepper sauce
Pinch of salt

Place the lentils and 1 cup of water in a small saucepan and bring to a boil over medium heat. Cover the pan, reduce the heat to low and simmer the lentils about 20 minutes, or until they are tender. Transfer the lentils and any remaining liquid to a food processor or blender and process until smooth. Add the remaining ingredients and process until smooth, scraping down the sides of the container with a rubber spatula as necessary. Transfer the dip to a small bowl and serve. Makes about 1 1/4 cups

Note: If red lentils are unavailable, another color may be used.

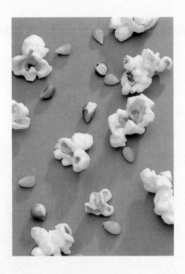

POPCORN WITH HERBED GOAT CHEESE

Drenching popcorn in butter adds lots of saturated fat and cholesterol to an otherwise high-fiber, low-calorie snack. By substituting a modest amount of relatively lowfat cheese, you consume more calcium and less fat.

CALORIES per serving	57
51% Carbohydrate	8 g
16% Protein	2 g
33% Fat	2 g
CALCIUM	4 mg
IRON	.3 mg
SODIUM	71 mg

3 tablespoons popcorn, approximately (about 3 cups popped)

1 ounce garlic-herb goat cheese
1 tablespoon chopped fresh parsley
1/4 teaspoon black pepper

Pop the corn in a hot-air popper. Meanwhile, heat the cheese in a large skillet over low heat, stirring constantly, until it melts. Add the popcorn, parsley and pepper to the skillet and toss quickly to combine. Makes 4 servings

Note: If garlic-herb goat cheese is unavailable, you can substitute 1 ounce of Neufchatel cheese blended with 1/4 teaspoon of chopped garlic and 1/2 teaspoon of dried herbs.

PINEAPPLE-COCONUT SHAKE

The pineapple and coconut in this shake add fiber, which conventional milk shakes lack.

CALORIES per serving	150
70% Carbohydrate	27 g
12% Protein	5 g
18% Fat	3 g
CALCIUM	154 mg
IRON	1 mg
SODIUM	142 mg

1/2 cup buttermilk
1 cup fresh pineapple chunks, or
1 cup juice-packed pineapple chunks, drained

1 tablespoon sweetened shredded coconut
1/2 teaspoon coconut extract

Place all of the ingredients in a blender and process for 5 to 10 seconds, or until blended. Pour the shake into a tall glass and serve. Makes 1 serving

STRAWBERRY-BANANA SHAKE

Strawberries, like all other berries, are a rich source of fiber. Recent reassessments of the dietary fiber content of foods show that strawberries contain twice as much fiber as previous measurements indicated.

CALORIES per serving	332
72% Carbohydrate	64 g
16% Protein	14 g
12% Fat	5 g
CALCIUM	443 mg
IRON	2 mg
SODIUM	162 mg

1 cup plain lowfat yogurt
3/4 cup fresh strawberries, washed and hulled, or 1 cup unsweetened frozen strawberries

1 medium-size banana, peeled
1 tablespoon wheat bran
2 teaspoons honey
2 ice cubes (optional)

Combine all of the ingredients in a blender and process, turning the machine on and off, for 5 to 10 seconds, or until the mixture is smooth and frothy. Pour the shake into a tall glass and serve.   Makes 1 serving

BLUEBERRY FRAPPE

This thick shake derives its texture not from ice cream but from wheat bran, one of the richest sources of dietary fiber.

CALORIES per serving	207
77% Carbohydrate	43 g
14% Protein	8 g
9% Fat	2 g
CALCIUM	229 mg
IRON	1 mg
SODIUM	203 mg

3/4 cup buttermilk
1 cup fresh or frozen blueberries
1 teaspoon grated lemon peel

1 tablespoon wheat bran
2 teaspoons honey
2 ice cubes

Combine all of the ingredients in a food processor or blender and process, turning the machine on and off, for 5 to 10 seconds, or until smooth and frothy. Pour the frappe into a tall glass and serve.   Makes 1 serving

CAROB MILK SHAKE

Loaded with fat and sugar, a regular chocolate milk shake can be a dietary disaster. This recipe, however, uses skim milk and cholesterol-lowering oat bran. The sweetness comes from the vanilla extract and the carob, which has a chocolaty taste.

CALORIES per serving	124
60% Carbohydrate	18 g
32% Protein	10 g
8% Fat	1g
CALCIUM	322 mg
IRON	.5 mg
SODIUM	132 mg

1 cup skim milk
1 tablespoon oat bran
2 teaspoons carob powder

1/2 teaspoon vanilla extract
2 ice cubes

Combine all the ingredients in a blender and process 5 to 10 seconds, or until smooth. Pour the shake into a tall glass and serve.   Makes 1 serving

PROP CREDITS

Cover: shorts—The Gap, San Francisco, Calif.; pages 25-27: sweat pants, sweat shirts—The Gap, San Francisco, Calif.; pages 32-45: sweat shirt—The Gap, San Francisco, Calif.; pages 50-71: sweat pants, shirt—Naturalife, New York City; pages 72-75: unitard —Dance France Ltd., Santa Monica, Calif.; pages 80-93: leotard —Dance France. Santa Monica, Calif.; page 94: sweat shirt—The Gap, San Francisco, Calif.; pages 98-119: sweat pants, shirt—The Gap, San Francisco, Calif.; pages 120-123: shirt—Calvin Klein Menswear, New York City, shorts—The Gap, San Francisco, Calif., shoes—Reebok International Ltd., Avon, Mass.; page 128: plate courtesy of Deborah Ragasto, Nyack, N.Y.; teapots—The Hall China Co., East Liverpool, Ohio, spoon—Platypus, New York City, tablecloth—Ad Hoc Softwares, New York City; page 129: bowl courtesy of Bonnie Slotnick, New York City; page 131: glasses—Platypus, New York City; page 132: plate—Mood Indigo, New York City; page 133: plate—Platypus, New York City, flatware—The Pottery Barn, New York City, napkin—Ad Hoc Softwares, New York City; page 134: plates, spoon—Mood Indigo, New York City, tablecloth —Pierre Deux, New York City; page 137: spoon courtesy of Nola Lopez, New York City; Page 139: tablecloth—Ad Hoc Softwares, New York City.

ACKNOWLEDGMENTS

All cosmetics and grooming products supplied by Clinique Labs, Inc., New York City

Off-camera warm-up equipment: rowing machine supplied by Precor USA, Redmond, Wash.; Tunturi stationary bicycle supplied by Amerec Corp., Bellevue, Wash.

Washing machine and dryer supplied by White-Westinghouse, Columbus, Ohio

Our thanks to the American Massage Therapy Association and Michael Yessis, Ph.D., of Sports Training, Inc., Escondido, Calif., for their research assistance

Index prepared by Ian Tucker

Production by Giga Communications

PHOTOGRAPHY CREDITS

All photographs by Steven Mays, Rebus, Inc.

ILLUSTRATION CREDITS

Pages 8-9, illustration: David Flaherty; page 11, illustration: David Flaherty; page 13, illustration: David Flaherty; page 14, illustration: David Flaherty; page 19, illustration: David Flaherty; page 21, chart: Brian Sisco and Tammy Colichio; page 23, chart: Brian Sisco and Tammy Colichio; page 97, illustration: Dana Burns.

INDEX